DHEAI'S MISSING LINK

ORIENTAL MEDICINE
&
EASTERN PHILOSOPHY

DHEAI ISSAID

To my Family, especially my Parents,

I am forever grateful for the wisdom and the knowledge you have bestowed upon me, all of which has enabled me to become the man I am today.

May God, Bless You in This Life and The Next

All my Love

Dheai

ACKNOWLEDGEMENTS

A very special thanks to EmmaJane O'Connell,
Florence Kati, Nina Kati & Dani Dunne, who supported
me and volunteered their time and expertise.

They worked tirelessly to make this book happen
and to make it happen in the best way possible.

A big massive thanks to you from the bottom
of my heart – I would have been lost without you!

Dheai.

DISCLAIMER

I am a General Oriental Practitioner: I am not a
licensed Medical Doctor.

I strongly encourage all to adhere to the strict instructions
prescribed by their licensed medical professionals.

NOTE TO THE READER:

This is Dheai's third book and it starts from Page 29,
the previous pages are from his first & second books,
'Oriental Medicine & Eastern Philosophy'

CONTENTS

INTRODUCTION

I write this introduction to the subjects of Oriental medicine, Eastern philosophy and Feng Shui in the hope that I can convey the importance of the powerful knowledge of the teachings contained within these pages. The book's author, Dheai Ilsaaid, and I work hard to empower others by sharing the secret science behind this philosophy through our work and through education. This book and the information contained within is not intended to disregard or replace modern medicine, and Dheai is not a medical doctor. However, it can be regarded as an alternative approach that can be used alongside modern medicine as a complement to general practice. As they say, ask the right person the right question at the right time and you will get the right answer – and maybe that answer (or part thereof) is right here waiting for you to discover it.

On reading this book bear in mind you may have been in a certain mind-set and emotional state at the time, so you were more likely to be engaged by specific topics as they grabbed you, because they may have held interest or value or relevance for you at that moment. However, each time you re-read this book, you will most likely discover new things, linking more and more of the information together to form a bigger picture as you go. This is what is most fascinating about these teachings – the pieces of information, the links that bring this information together into segments, how the linked segments connect, and then the big picture itself. It will stretch your mind and open it to new possibilities. And this is not just a book for now, to be discarded and disposed of later, but it is ideal as a quick leaf-through, to fully re-read, to use as a reference manual, to share with others, and to pass on to the next generation for their benefit.

It is important for me to mention here that this philosophy is completely independent of religion, nor does it matter what the reader's beliefs are or what their value system is. This philosophy is a universal approach that does not depend on a person's age, sex, colour, creed, nationality, background or experiences. This information is self-empowering.

It is a new philosophy and a new way of living. It may be that you are looking to educate yourself in this area, or perhaps to find a solution to a specific health issue, but in any case, for you this may be a completely new perspective as well as a totally new subject, and I want to help you grasp the reasoning behind this philosophy in the easiest way possible. I have studied under Dheai Ilsaaid so that my knowledge could become more full spectrum, and I often recommend him to me clients to ensure a totally holistic approach to their wellbeing. In descriptive terms, I deal with the Feng Shui of the home and Dheai deals with the Feng Shui of the body. Ultimately, the goal of Eastern philosophy is to create balance in mind, body and soul. My recommendations combined with Dheai's treatments, mean clients can get better health more quickly, thereby impacting their lives in an even more powerful way.

Dheai's background and studies in Oriental medicine and Eastern philosophy have led him on a fascinating journey and immersed him in learning for many years – knowledge that has been passed down to him through generations which he is keen to share with the world today. Dheai has extensive training in deep acupuncture, Reiki, massage, iridology, cranial sacral manipulation, medical yoga, and much more. He treats all ailments, the most common being insomnia, depression, arthritis, infertility, obesity, respiratory issues and illnesses such as high blood pressure and diabetes. Dheai used many techniques to diagnose his clients health issues based on Yin and Yang and the five elements, such as facial diagnosis, tongue diagnosis and pulse diagnosis, and he also employs techniques to treat the sub-conscious mind, including positive affirmations, neuron-linguistic programming, mindfulness, meditation, timeline therapy, dream interpretation, hypnosis, and beyond the physical body to an astral level by accessing the soul and spirit. When Dheai diagnoses a client, he uses certain indicators to determine their health issues, and then he selects the best treatment specific to them. This includes diet and advice on nutritional needs, a course of acupuncture treatments to redress imbalances, exercises to improve postural alignment affecting stance and gait, and specific types of physical movements that retain the human mind to break bad habits and to positively affect the sub-conscious mind.

THE FUNDAMENTALS

Breath, The Life Force

Let me begin by explaining in plain language the fundamentals of this philosophy so that the content herein is put into a simple format with a logical framework. I want to make it easier for you, the reader, to understand health holistically from an oriental perspective. Breathing is top priority in Oriental medicine. Everything is based on breathing, that is breathing properly, and this is entirely the foundation for your good health, because this is the basis for the life force

Breathing is life and life is breathing. Your immune system starts at the nose, because this is where the chi first enters the body. Breathing in and out through the nose allows the air to be filtered and regulated before it enters the body. It is the breath that carries oxygen to all parts of the body, so this chi must enter and exit the body properly to nourish the organs correctly and, also, to positively affect the mind and the emotions.

Inhaling is Yin and nourishing. Exhaling is Yang and about letting go and moving on. Oxygen represents life and inherited genes. Carbon dioxide represents death. There must be a good balance of both for a happy, healthy life.

The act of inhalation is to breathe air into the lungs properly, bringing oxygen and nourishment to all the organs. The act of exhaling is to release carbon and other gaseous toxins from the body. This directly affects many systems and organ functions in the body; digestion, excretion, fertilisation and so on. If breathing is not carried out properly and effectively, then this will lead to many health issues, e.g., constipation. Everything depends on the breath to function correctly, including non-physical senses such as concentration, memorisation, anticipation, perception, wisdom, intuition and intellect.

As part of Oriental medicine, treatment begins with learning how to breathe properly, positively affecting and changing the chi in the body, thereby changing the thoughts, emotions, behaviours, and overall health of the person. The body's temperature will regulate, they will begin to feel calm, their memory recall improves, and they will have better mental clarity, amongst many other immediate benefits.

Cause & Effect, Action & Consequence

This philosophy is about cause and effect, action and consequence. Using it to good effect will result in a positive outcome due to several factors; your thoughts, your behaviour, the consequences. The way you perceive things and your perspective on everything can be affected by this knowledge, and therefore the subsequent decisions you make. Your actions that is the way you behave, can also be affected including changing your learned habits. Furthermore, your thoughts and actions have a karmic impact too, i.e., the consequence. These karmic vibrations affect your mind, body, spirit and the rest of the universe, and negative or positive thoughts and actions will lead to opposite results. By doing good deeds you will generate goodwill – what goes around will come around, no matter the fact that it may happen at a different time and from a different source, but it will come, and it will come at the right time.

Karma is also affected by the law of physics; in that the reverberation of your actions will have as much effect on you as it will for the person whom you are affecting or the situation that you are bringing about. In Feng Shui terms everything we do in our lifetime affects up to seven generations that come after us.

Simultaneously, during our lifetime up to seven generations are looking after us from 'above'. This is cause and effect, action and consequence. Life is a wheel that is always turning, and this wheel of life eventually goes back to its starting point. For instance, when we are born our eyesight has yet to be developed, we cannot walk, we have little comprehension or ability to remember, and we have no teeth to chew our food. If we live for long enough, our sight will totally diminish, we will have great difficulty walking, we will begin to lose our cognitive and retentive functions, and even our teeth will eventually fall out. Not pretty, I know, but this is the natural order of things! Once your thoughts and actions become more positive, then the consequence of this is positive change in your life as well as for those whom you are connected to, and in turn this will improve your luck, your health will be good, your relationships will become better, you will have more support in your life and you will have a greater sense of wellbeing – these are your fortunate blessings in life. As they say, it is much better to be born lucky then wealthy...

Health consists of all aspects of the self; your mind both conscious and subconscious, your structural and functioning body, your spirit and soul that resides within. In fact, every aspect of how you are made at a cellular level from the beginnings of humankind to the way you function, including your emotional health starting from its true beginnings, i.e., from even before you were born (your inherited emotions which make up your emotional DNA that links you to your lineage), to the energy imprint you will leave behind when you depart this life.

Oriental medicine and Eastern philosophy is truly and completely holistic and affects all aspects of your wellbeing, and all those connected to you, across many generations before and after your physical existence, because we are all as one, existing as one and even resonating as one at a similar frequency to the planet, and the rest of the plants and creatures that inhabit Earth. The energy frequency of the vibration of the individual and of the collective whole relates to the entire Cosmos. This philosophy is a universal approach to life and death, the whole universe, and on into the afterlife.

Timing

To determine a person's health at a specific moment in time, this holistic approach is used to read the energy flow (also referred to as prana or chi) within a person as well as the energetic imprint that is carried forward from generations prior which affects their mind, body, spirit and soul, and then clients are treated accordingly. This is because energy is constantly moving and changing, therefore the treatment of a person's health will be entirely different during their next visit to the practitioner. This is a new moment and now their situation is different again. In this way, the diagnosis of a person's health on each occasion must be freshly addressed, and therefore their treatment is adjusted accordingly, just as the timing in my clients' lives will be different each time I visit their homes to carry out an assessment of their Feng Shui. Timing is vital in Oriental medicine, Eastern philosophy and Feng Shui. There are lots of different timings, but one example is that there are energy channels in the body that convert from Yin to Yang every two hours through a 24-hour time cycle. This is like an up and down, peak and through process that has many implications, including which organ belongs to each 2-hour time slot, and how they are affected during that period. If in pain, the form of pain you will feel will also change accordingly, e.g., throbbing, scalding, shooting, stabbing, burning, or piercing pain. Endorphins, the body's natural response to pain, will significantly reduce at night, and then the pain will become more intense. The time slot 2 hours before sunrise is the most intense of all when a mini explosion of cosmic energy takes place in the universe. This is when the Cosmos is at its most active, and therefore it is the most ideal time to attempt to conceive a child. It is at night time when the body must rest and rejuvenate as this is when cells are repaired or replaced, and when the mind empties to allow the brain to take in new information. It is for this reason that it is so important for a person to sleep well at night especially during specific 2-hour time slots in the 24-hour cycle. If you miss this opportunity to rest the mind and body, then no matter when you try to catch up at other times in the 24-hour time cycle, whether a short nap or longer, you will only snooze without sleeping well and still feel tired when you wake. This is detrimental to the sub-conscious mind and to the body itself, negatively impacting on a person's health.

Finally

May I take this opportunity to thank Dheai most sincerely for being my mentor, my confidant, my teacher and my friend, and for inviting me to write the foreword for this, his first book. It has been a long and enjoyable journey, and I am most grateful for the teachings I have received from the many wonderful people I was blessed to meet along the way. New, the next destination on this fascinating journey is just as exciting. I hope you will enjoy reading this book, and by learning the science behind Oriental medicine, Eastern philosophy and Feng Shui, I also hope these teachings will help you to live an extraordinary life and truly shine.

Nina Kati

Introduction by Nina Kati, © 2017

DHEAI'S MISSING LINK

ORIENTAL MEDICINE
&
EASTERN PHILOSOPHY

LETTER

Dear Reader,

This is a very important notice, so I ask for your full attention before you go any further with this book. Please keep in mind, English is not my first language, so I may write in a way that is somewhat different than the reader is accustomed to.

Throughout this book you will encounter many terms, one such term is *'Muslim'*, this is to provide the reader with an understanding of my background and upbringing, both of which have been very important in leading me to gain the knowledge I now hold of Oriental Medicine and Philosophy. Also, it is important that you the reader, understand the teachings within this book have travelled down through many generations, each generation has passed on its wisdom to the next, as I now try to do for you.

I must be clear; it is not my intention or that of this book, to promote or encourage any change within the readers own belief system. Throughout this book, the wisdom of several world religions will appear in the text, just as I would never try to promote my faith to the reader nor is it my intention to promote the faith of any other world religion. Within the history and culture of humanity, veins of wisdom and messages of healing flow, while one piece of wisdom may originate within Christianity, this does not mean one must be a Christian to understand or appreciate it.

During my Yoga training, the class, myself included, all received literature on the teachings of Buddhism, it was not the intention of our teacher to try and convert us, but merely it was to increase our knowledge and understanding of the art of Yoga. Your personal beliefs are your own, my clinic, my lectures and my book are open to all, my door will never close to you, we are all human beings and as such should treat one another with love and respect.

Middle Eastern Philosophy dates back over 7000 years, the labels society have stuck upon us all, are just labels, the teachings and wisdom from all our forefathers, are no less pure today than they were 7000 years ago.

Best Wishes,

    Dheai Ilsaaid.

The first three chapters of this book cover the same introductory material as the first three chapters of the first book. The reason for this is self-explanatory for first time readers and returning readers may need a refresher on the foundations

Let's Recap for Some

&

Begin Anew for Others

(Skip To Part 4 if You are Confident)

PART 1

FREQUENTLY ASKED QUESTIONS.

Q1: Could you please tell me what Oriental Medicine means?

Oriental Medicine means treating the patient as a human being and not just treating the symptoms they present with when they come to the clinic. The patient is treated holistically, from every aspect.

Q2: What are these aspects?

In Oriental Medicine, the human being is studied from the following aspects:

- ❖ Structurally: The physical make-up of the body.
- ❖ Functionally: How the body works and how each organ works individually.
- ❖ Psychologically: What type of character the patient has.
- ❖ Emotionally: How the clients behave and react to fluctuating emotions.
- ❖ Mentally: The ability for productive thinking and behavior.
- ❖ Sexually: The sexual desire and sexual motivation

Q3: When you talk about structurally, how are these human systems and organs formed?

They are formed when a new human being is created, in other words, during pregnancy. When the sperm meets the ova, this announces the start of new life, and the development process takes place during the pregnancy. Within the developing baby, new tissue is created and organs are formed. Different organs combine to form different systems, for example, the stomach is part of the digestive system. The stages of development are cell, tissue organ, system and baby.

Q4: Could you explain to me about cells?

A cell is a unique individual entity, which forms every aspect in the universe, this means every aspect in the universe contains cells, and the cell divides into two parts, the plus and the minus, or the Yin and the Yang. Seventy per cent of every cell is made up of water - no water - no cell, no cell - no life. Each cell has its unique brain, which controls the cell's activity and function in the human body. This means the activity that determines the life span of the cell, the production of the cell, the wastes that the cell produces and the regeneration of the cell. All these activities are connected to the brain and the heart.

Q5: In Oriental Medicine, what gives the energy to the cell?

Qi (Chi) is the life force of every living thing in the universe. Just as different cells have different functions in the body, so also are their different types of Qi, relating to the different organs and their function. There is Yin Qi and Yang Qi. I will discuss Yin and Yang later.

Q6: What form can Qi take?

Qi could be material or non-material; substantial or non-substantial; tangible or non-tangible; visible or non-visible; dense or hollow.

Q7: What can affect the Qi in the body?

Qi can be affected by deficiency or excess as well as rebelliousness or collapse. For example, Lung Qi deficiency over a long period can lead to shallow breathing and asthma. The excess over a long period can be like a traffic jam. It causes restriction which in turn may cause a tumour. Qi can be rebellious, for example, if it doesn't follow its correct path in the body. Rebellious stomach Qi causes the flow to go upwards instead of downwards resulting in vomiting. The collapse of Qi occurs when things are not held in place, like prolapse or haemorrhoids. I will give a very simple example of Qi (energy). At one of my lectures about Oriental Medicine, one member of the audience was from a medical background. He asked if I dissected your leg, would I see this Qi that you are explaining? When I told him that Qi is non-visible, he asked how people could be expected to believe in something they can't see. I explained that this is the difference between the study of Western and Oriental Medicine. You can't see oxygen or the air, but you know it is there. You can't see the air, but if you move your hand quickly in front of you, you can feel the movement of the air. This is the interaction of Qi and the transformation of Qi from something non-visible to something you can feel. In the same way, if you dissect an electric cable, you can see the small electrical wires inside of it, but you won't be able to physically see the flow of the electricity (the plus and the) inside those wires you won't be able to see this electricity until the light is switched on. This is the interaction of the Yin Qi with the Yang Qi, in other words, the interaction of the positive and the negative.

Keep an open mind and look at things from every perspective, see how people in different parts of the world view things. In the Middle, East Qi is regarded as a force from God. Every living matter contains energy, and this energy is called Qi. Different countries have different names for it. In India, from a yoga perspective, Qi is called Prana, the life force and the Power of the Breath. There is oneness in the Universe. We all breathe the same oxygen. The air, the oxygen, all on earth was created by God. We all share the products of the earth, and we all return to the earth whether we have belief or not. As we have established, Qi can be visible or non-visible whether from an Oriental or Western Perspective.

Q8: How does all this apply to me when I attend for treatment?

As we mentioned earlier, Qi is a force, power or energy. When Qi moves, it moves the blood (circulation). Movement is regarded as Yang (heat), while blood is Yin (cold) because it is liquid. When you run, you feel warm because Qi is moving the blood. The blood must nourish the muscles so that they can do the action. We refer to this as the blood nourishing the Qi. If a patient complains of cold hands and cold feet, this means they have a Yang deficiency (lack of heat). This lack of heat will lead to the stagnation of blood. Over a long period, this stagnation can lead to various circulation problems, such as varicose veins or puffy swollen ankles or clots. In the clinic, we check your tongue and pulse to find out what imbalance in your body is contributing to your complaint. Treatment involves a combination of acupuncture, dietary advice and exercises such as Kundalini yoga, and the patient is treated from every aspect as I mentioned earlier, emotionally, physically, etc.

Q9: How can this be done with needles and exercise?

Treatment is done per the pathology of Qi, in other words, what has gone wrong with Qi. If there is a deficiency, Qi needs to be regulated. If there is excess, Qi needs to be decreased. If Qi is rebellious, it needs to be restored to its correct flow. If Qi is stagnant, it must be moved. Take Lung Qi deficiency for example. If lung energy is weak, there will be shallow breathing, leading to asthma. The whole body will pay the price for the weakness of one organ. The patient will start to feel tired because the whole body isn't getting enough oxygen. During treatment, we will tune the lungs as an organ, and the body in general.

Headache can be an example of excess. When Qi is not moving, it can block the affected channels of the body. We treat this by decreasing the excess in the affected channel to restore the balance. Later I will talk about the six forms of headache, as seen from an oriental perspective.

Qi can be rebellious, for example in the stomach. It can cause food to flow back up, instead of following the correct downward direction for digestion. We treat this by directing the Qi back into the stomach channel. We also tonify the spleen, as these two organs work together in oriental medicine. Stagnation of Qi can lead to stagnation of blood and tissue, for example, fibroids. We treat this by moving Qi. In the case of fibroids, we treat the woman's period and reproductive system. We focus on the circulation and hormones and will treat the liver channel, as this is the meridian, which passes through the reproductive system.

Qi can be said to sink, for example in cases of prolapse, miscarriage or piles. This means that Qi is weak and is not able to keep the tissue and the organ in place. In this case, we push Qi upwards and tone the organ and channel and everything else involved with fluid or lymph or blood. In Oriental Medicine, the practitioner can be described as the driver. The needles are the steering. Qi is petrol. The channels are the roads. The practitioner directs the energy where it is most needed, the driver steers the wheels in the direction he wants to go to.

Q10: Is there only one type of Qi?

We are born with Constitutional Qi, which we inherit from our parents. It is called the Pre-Heaven Qi. From an oriental point of view, it relates to the kidneys. It represents DNA, the genetic material we inherit from our parents. This Qi depends on our parents' age and health at the time of our conception, as well as the parents' physical and emotional state during pregnancy and delivery. We can't increase our Pre-Heaven Qi, but we can maintain it by looking after our health in general. A further type of Qi is Post-Heaven Qi. This can be maintained and improved by the air we breathe, the food we eat, maintaining a healthy lifestyle, sleeping, exercising, and having a positive mental attitude. What we know in western medicine as the immune system is known as Wei Qi in oriental medicine. It surrounds the surface of our skin, and protects against any pathogenic invaders, like bacteria or viruses. Nutritive Qi is deeper inside the body's organs. It carries nutrients to the cells and moves the waste products. Equivalent to interstitial fluid.

Breathe, Deep Breath, Breathe

PART 2

YIN & YANG

Yin and Yang are the foundation of our universe, the foundation of us as living beings. Life starts from a single male cell (sperm = Yin) and the single female cell (ovum = Yang).

Yin is the fluid aspect of evthing. Its function in the human body is to cool and moisturize and nourish the cells and organs. I speak about cytoplasm. This is the fluid that cells float in, and without fluid, the cells will die. Blood is fluid. Yin is a portion of blood, and blood is a portion of Yin. They share the same functions, cooling, moisturizing, and nourishing the cells.

Yang represents the warming and the pushing upwards activities, such as circulation. Hence, Yin needs Yang. Yin is fluid in nature, Yang is movement or energy or Qi. Yin nourishes the Yang, just as blood nourishes the Qi. The Qi pushes blood in the circulation of everything — fluids, lymph, blood, and the vital substances in the body. When you hear the saying "cold hands, warm heart", you are talking about circulation or the movement of blood as Yin.

Yang is activity. It pushes and warms and moves. Yin is the resting state. While you are sitting reading this book, your heart is beating 70 or 80 beats per minute. You are in a resting or Yin state.

When you go for a walk or a run, you are using muscular activity. This activity needs fuel so that the muscles can sustain the activity. The heart is a pump. It is a muscular organ. It has a Yang job to do. It pumps blood to the working muscles to carry on the activity of pushing and moving. The heart must raise its rate to supply enough oxygen to the cells. The faster you run, the faster the heartbeats, the warmer you start to feel because Yang is heat and movement.

Oxygen is Yin in nature. It is carried in the blood. As I said earlier, blood is the portion of Yin, and Yin is the portion of blood. Both are fluid, which cools and moisturizes. When the body starts to overheat during activity, it starts to produce toxins like urine and lactic acid because of the build-up of carbon dioxide. CO_2 is Yang in nature. The body tries to protect itself; therefore, you start to sweat to remove the toxins through your skin, which is the largest organ in the body. From an Oriental point of view, the lungs are closely related to the skin. I will deal with this later, but basically, the skin supports the lungs and the lungs support the skin by releasing toxins in the sweat to decrease the pressure on the lungs and heart during muscular activity.

Yang is activity, activity produces heat. Yin is cold and wet. It is associated with resting. Yang is fast while Yin is slow. Now we can look at Yin and Yang from a western perspective. What makes the heart beat faster as you start running, and what will decide the amount of oxygen and glucose required to be released at the time of running? What will decide where the oxygen and glucose go, to which working muscle? From a western perspective, the brain must control these functions. Yin and Yang are involved from an Oriental Perspective.

Our emotional state can also affect the heartbeat and circulation. The sympathetic nervous system is Yang because it speeds the heart rate and circulation, and speeds the release of hormones and glucose. This is what happens when we feel joy or happiness or excitement. The sympathetic nervous system is also involved when we talk about fight or flight, for example when we run away from danger. The parasympathetic nervous system is the opposite. It is Yin in nature. It slows things down. It slows the heart rate, slows the oxygen supply, and stops releasing hormones, etc.

We need to be clear when we talk about Yin and Yang and give as many examples as possible from a western perspective. It's not only during an activity that the heart raises its beat and rhythm. You might be resting (Yin) but may feel your heart is beating fast. There may be an infection in the body. The immune system is Yin in nature. It is there in the body all the time but is dormant until it is activated when required.

The lymphatic system is Yang in nature because the lymph must keep moving all the time, to protect the body whether there is an infection in the body or not. As a substance, blood is Yin (fluid), but it is Yang activity /movement. When blood moves, it carries everything that is required by the body, fluids, nutrients, etc. Blood carries red blood cells which are Yin in nature. It also carries white blood cells which are Yang in nature. We know that Yang rises. White blood cells are Yang but they should not be raised without reason. The body's white blood cell count rises when there is an infection. The white blood cells outnumber the red from an Oriental perspective. The Yang consumes the Yin. The person may look pale and tired and they may have a temperature. If the patient's immune system (Wei Qi) is strong and there is no stagnation in the body, the patient may recover with no treatment either Western or Oriental.

But if the Wei Qi is weak, the following may occur:

When bacteria enter the body, they are active and multiply rapidly. A virus can remain dormant in the body for a period, just waiting to activate. A virus is Yin in nature because it is less active, and our body can adjust to it. Bacterial infections are more acute and must be dealt with immediately. In western medicine, antibiotics are commonly used to battle bacteria. Bacteria attack the body suddenly and do not have enough time to hide and read the immune system to deceive it. The immune system is your army and the pathogen is the enemy's army. It is very easy to pull the Yang down fast but it takes a longer time to nourish the Yin.

Regardless of what treatment the patient seeks the respiratory system is divided into two parts, the upper respiratory tract, and the lower respiratory tract. The upper consists of the nose, mouth, sinuses, throat, and tonsils. The lower consists of the trachea, bronchi, bronchioles, alveoli, lungs, diaphragm, and intercostal muscles.

In the first part of an attack by a pathogenic invader i.e. bacteria or virus, the Wei Qi/immune system engages in battle. If the Wei Qi is strong, it wins the battle and drives away the invader before it descends to the lower respiratory tract. This may be when the person has a cold with a slight cough, runny nose with white discharge, runny eyes, slight headache, slight temperature, and sore throat.

Your tonsils play a big part in stopping the invader from descending to the lower respiratory tract. They are the first part of our inner immune system. This explains why if a person has had his or her tonsils removed, they are more open to infection. If the immune system is very weak at the time of the attack, the infection can develop into a cough with green or yellow mucus, headache with high temperature, fast pulse, sweating, very sore and hot throat, fatigue, no energy, and no appetite. There may be a metallic taste in the mouth. All these are signs of Yang rising and consuming the Yin.

Our role as Oriental practitioners is to bring the balance back to the body, especially the respiratory, immune, and lymphatic systems.

PART 3

DAILY PRACTICAL EXAMPLES OF YIN AND YANG

This is a continuation of the application of the Yin and Yang from a bodily perspective and everything related to the universe and the following list. It will give a familiar day-to-day activity for the entire universe and for the human who lives in this universe. This means this is the interaction between the human and the universe and the universe and the human. This indicates the oneness of everything. Now if I want to continue listing, the list would be endless but I will give a couple of examples, which are related to all of us not only from a medical perspective but also as a human being.

Per the Yin and Yang theory, every Yin organ has a Yang job to do, and every Yang organ has a Yin job to do. For example, sperm is Yin because it is fluid. But the activity of the sperm is Yang. The sperm must move to reach the ova for fertilization. Movement is activity, and as we know, activity is Yang.

Female is Yin. The female breast tissue is dense, which means they are regarded as Yin. But the activity of the breast is Yang, due to the movement of the breast milk to supply nutrients for the baby. I will discuss the process of lactation later when I talk about how the woman's emotional state can affect the body's functions. The uterus is a hollow organ, so it is Yang. However, it has a Yin job to do which is to carry and hold the baby during pregnancy.

YIN	YANG
Female	Male
Night	Day
Water	Fire
Cold	Hot
Slow	Fast
Wet	Dry
Old	Young
Blood	Chi
Virus	Bacteria
Plant	Animal
Chronic	Acute
Sperm	Ova
Rest	Active
Visible	Invisible

NIGHT & DAY

Night is Yin, it is a time of rest and inactivity, and it is dark. The moon provides some light but not the heat and light of the sun. Daytime is Yang because it is a time of activity and movement. It's time for the sun to rise which is heat which is Yang. In the human body, a toothache can flare up in the night. The teeth are dense so they are Yin but their function (chewing) is Yang. The activity of chewing by day can consume the Yin, so there might not be enough Yin left to provide cooling pain relief. The stomach is a hollow organ so it is Yang, but it has a Yin job to do in producing gastric enzymes for digestion. Therefore, it's not a good idea to eat after 6 pm or late at night as the Yin is already used up during the day's digestive activity. The stomach Yin is no longer able to cool and moisturize so conditions like stomach ulcers or irritable bowel can flare up at night.

FIRE & WATER

Per the theory of Yin and Yang, Yin is water and Yang is fire. Fire means heat, water means cold. If you light a fire, it heats and rises upward. If you pour water, it cools and descends downwards. Illnesses such as stroke, tinnitus, and detached retina affect the head or face. They are all Yang conditions because as we know Yang rises. They are excess conditions but they may be based on a deficiency of Yin.

Dry irritated itchy eyes are Yang excess conditions but are based on a deficiency of Yin which is unable to complete the cooling and moisturizing function. In other words, the tear ducts are not producing sufficient lubricant thus resulting in the symptoms described. As always, the job of the Oriental Practitioner is to restore the balance between Yin and Yang. If there is too much water (Yin) in the body, this can lead to excess cold. This leads to Yang deficiency, as both Yin and Yang can consume the other. The ideal situation is one of balance.

HOT & COLD

Summer is hot. Heat is Yang. Winter is cold. Cold is Yin. Some conditions improve or worsen per the time of year. Some asthmatics find that their condition worsens when the weather is damp or cold. This leads to the accumulation of dampness and fluid in the body. It can turn into mucus and phlegm and obstruct the lungs. Rheumatoid arthritis is a Yang condition. The sufferer has signs of heat, such as swollen hot joints. When the person moves, the condition gets worse. Movement is activity, which produces further heat. It's like adding fuel to the fire. The patient feels better when at rest. The hot weather in the summertime can worsen the symptoms.

Osteoarthritis is different. It is a cold condition. It is defined as degeneration of the affected joint and is a sign of stagnation of Qi and blood. Qi pushes the blood to nourish andwarm the body, and carry waste from the cells. When Qi is stagnant it does not move the blood, so there is a cold condition. Therefore, sufferers of osteoarthritis find that their condition is worse in the winter. They are also usually worse first thing in the morning, because of the inactivity of resting. The symptoms get worse when the person is at rest, but once they start to move, the heat of movement helps relieve the symptoms. Movement is Yang. Yang produces heat. Heat moves the blood to warm and moisturize and nourish the joints and everything connected to them like the ligaments and tendons etc. Yin and Yang conditions also relate to human conditions both mentally and psychologically. Most mental and psychological problems are related to the heart from an Oriental Perspective.

YIN AND YANG DIRECTION OF FLOW

Yang rises upwards. All the Yang channels meet in the face and head. Conditions such as tinnitus, headache, migraine, itchy irritated eyes, and cataracts, are related to excess Yang. They might be based on blood deficiency or Yin deficiency or stagnation of Qi in the head or face. Yin moves downwards, water only flows in a downward direction. This explains why gout is a Yin condition. It mainly affects the big toes where the spleen channel starts from one side and the liver channel starts from the other side.

WET & DRY

Yin is wet and cold. If a person consumes a lot of cold or greasy food or lives in a damp cold environment, they may end up with conditions of Yang deficiency, Spleen Yang deficiency, or Kidney Yang deficiency.

Yang deficiency can allow damp and fluids to accumulate in the lower legs, especially in the muscles and ankles, which may swell and look very puffy. Sometimes the person may have difficulty walking or doing ordinary daily activity. The best way to clear the dampness and fluid and help the lower leg circulation is for the person to try non-impact activities such as swimming or cycling or Yoga and Pilates. Any movement, which involves raising the legs or the joints will help. If the person is overweight, losing weight would help to get rid of damp and fluids.

Dryness is a Yang condition. It is based on Yin deficiency or blood deficiency. Both Yin and blood cool and moisturize the tissues of the organs. This explains why patients with anemia may suffer from constipation. There may not be enough blood to cool and moisturize the bowel. Dryness can affect any part of the body, especially the stomach, bowel, and skin.

VISIBLE & NON-VISIBLE

Yin is described as material, substantial, visible, and tangible. It is dense. Water is Yin. You can see it and touch it. Yang is non-material, non-substantial, non-visible, and intangible. Heat is Yang. You can't see it or touch it. However, if you heat a bowl of water the water turns into steam. This is the transitional stage between water being material and non-material. When the water evaporates, you can no longer see it or feel it. The heat has caused the water to evaporate. Yang has consumed the Yin. The sun's heat on the oceans and lakes and rivers causes evaporation. The clouds formed to meet with hot or cold air, causing rain, which starts the cycle all over again. Water can quench fire as Yin can consume Yang. All this relates to the five elements.

FAST & SLOW

Per the Yin and Yang theory, a rapid or fast pulse is a sign of excess. This means excess heat whether it is based on excess or deficiency or is caused by interior or exterior conditions. A fast walk or run speeds up the heart rate. This leads to sweating. Sweating is a sign of excess heat. During the process of sweating the body is protecting itself by eliminating toxins like urea, lactic acid, and salt. A slow sluggish pulse can be a sign of weak circulation. Inactivity produces a slow pulse because of a lack of cardiovascular activity. The pulse can appear to sink deep down and can be hard to find. The person may be cold most of the time, mainly in the hands and feet. A person with low blood pressure may have a pulse that is weak and slow.

OLD AGE & YOUTH

Old age is regarded as Yin. Yin is rest. The older we get the less active we become. Our metabolic rate slows down as we age. As we know, activity is heat. Older people tend to have a weaker circulation which explains why they feel the cold more. They prefer peace, quiet, and calm most of the time. Some may also speak more quietly. Some of them spend their time reading or watching TV. These activities are done at rest. All these are signs of Yin and are the opposite of the activity and movement of Yang.

Youth is regarded as Yang and activity. The more we develop during adolescence, the stronger our body gets. Our skeletal and muscular systems grow. In adolescence, we are more emotional and we rush into things with little or no thought for the consequences. Our sympathetic nervous system speeds everything up and controls most of the youth stage. Our physical development is faster than our mental development. Hormones are flowing, which makes it easy to fall in love or to end a relationship.

This is particularly true for boys as boys are Yang and girls are Yin. Yang is speed. Yin is slow and rest. That also explains why women are slower to start relationships, especially after a previous breakup. The longer a relationship goes on, the greater the impact when it ends. That's what people mean when they say 'my heart is broken'. Later I will explain this in more detail from an Oriental Perspective.

Talking about youth and old age, men and women differ, but the physical decline of the body and the hormones are the same, regardless of where they come from. As the woman has menopause the man has also a different form of menopause. As women age their oestrogen level drops. As we know from an Oriental Perspective, oestrogen is the Yin aspect of the woman and the Yin must cool and moisturize.

When the oestrogen level drops vastly women experience the following menopausal symptoms:

1. Feeling hot most of the time especially during the night. Having hot flushes, which can happen at any time of the day, but mainly at night because the night is Yin and the daytime is Yang.
2. Night sweats. There is a difference between daytime sweating and night sweating and there is a difference between sweating without activity or with activity or sweating with a normal temperature or due to an infection. Later I will explain the heart from an Oriental Perspective, sweating is related to the heart.
3. Restless and irritable, with anger, worry, and anxiety.
4. Difficulty sleeping, e.g. if you are not able to fall asleep in the first place this is related to your blood, and if you fall asleep easily but wake up easily and you cannot go back to sleep again, and you think and most of your thinking is negative and expecting the worst and creating your scenario which will include the following questions, 'how, what, when and why' and you get no answer and you keep living in this vicious circle, this is related to the mind and the mind is connected to the heart from an Oriental perspective.
5. Constipation
6. Craving of sugar
7. Itchy irritant and dry eyes

8. Lack of memory, weak concentration and focus, a lack mental clarity and sharpness
9. Lack of sexual desire

What we have already said about women can be applied to men but men have a different hormone which, as you know, is called testosterone. When the testosterone level drops, a man will have the following symptoms in addition to what I mentioned earlier about the woman.

1. Weak back, all the back, and spine in general but especially the lower back
2. Frequent urination
3. Lack of motivation or physical energy
4. Baldness, hair falling out, either completely or in a specific area, later I will explain how the location of the bald spot is related to a certain channel, organ, and emotion.
5. Getting angry or upset for the slightest reason. Later when I talk about the kidney from a five-element perspective, I will explain in more detail why some men or women have either excessive sexual desire with no contentment or satisfaction, or women may not be able to reach orgasm or climax. A man may have impotence or be unable to maintain the erection or have premature ejaculation from a western perspective.

SUMMER & WINTER

Summer is Yang because Yang is heat, heat comes from the sun, the sun itself is Yang because the sun rises in the daytime, daytime is activity. Also, the sun sends the light, light is Yang, dark is Yin. Winter is cold with wet, damp and rain, all these are signs of Yin, the moon comes out at night because the night itself is Yin because Yin is rest when people go to bed to sleep. The light from the moon, is different from the light from the sun. It is a Yin light because it does not have the type of heat the sun has, it has a different job and function which influence the world and all the environment in general, it influences the weather and the seasons.

CHRONIC & ACUTE

Per the Yin and Yang theory, a chronic condition means a condition that you have over a long period, which leads to demolishing the Yin. You know by now that Yin cools and moisturizes. The Yin can be demolished for various reasons:

1. A chronic sickness
2. Born with a hereditary disease or hereditary condition
3. Lack of rest, or sleep over a long period, varies from person to person per their physical capacity and the constitutional strength they were born with.
4. Use of medication over a long period is another reason for the demolition of the Yin, use of steroids, cortisone, alcohol will lead to the demolition of the Yin. This applies to our body but especially the organ which is connected to the substance that is being consumed, for example alcohol damages the liver, smoke damages the lungs, cholesterol, and fatty foods damage the heart. Any form of addiction whether heroin or cocaine will destroy the heart and the blood, and in turn will damage all the body from every aspect. Like smoke demolishes the lung Yin, which leads to dryness, and in some cases, it causes cancer, because the

Yin is the fluid aspect of the lungs that fills the pleural cavity.

5. Demolishing of the Yin will affect every joint. As you say in Ireland to make a long story short, you do not wake up in the morning and the doctor decides for you that you need a knee or hip replacement, or you don't sleep and you wake up the next day to have a stomach ulcer. This means the condition is there for a long time which caused the cartilage or the ligament or the fluid of the knee joint to be damaged.

6. If we exclude any physical injury, accident, car accident, or skiing accident, you don't need to have a Yin deficiency to have a knee or hip replacement. This is a different story. Walking, standing, sitting, running, or jogging in the wrong way will damage the joint and in turn, it will demolish the Yin of all the body especially the affected joint. The human posture contributes to the condition with which the clients present themselves at the clinic.

The acute condition covers the following criteria:

- ➢ Sudden
- ➢ Sharp
- ➢ Intense

It comes and goes like a wave either at regular intervals or at a specific time or a specific movement the person makes. For example, sciatica - the sciatic nerve passes from the lower back, back down to the back of the knee. If the nerve is pinched due to a compression of the vertebra or due to a massive strain to the muscles of the lower back this will lead to a shooting pain traveling down to the back of the leg with or without movement.

Some clients describe it as stabbing pain and the pain is not there all the time, it comes and goes.

From an Oriental perspective, this is regarded as an acute condition but if it is not being treated it will lead to a chronic condition that demolishes the Yin of all the body but especially the kidney and the bladder Yin as organs. The list of chronic and acute conditions is endless from an Oriental and Western Perspective.

ANIMALS & PLANTS

Per the Yin and Yang theory animals are regarded as Yang because animals move by either walking, running, flying, or swimming. Regardless of what movements animals make, they are regarded as Yang, because Yang is activity. The other reason is that the animals have a certain amount of intellect, but their intellect is different from human intellect their intellect matches the way that they are created. This means their intellect is related to their survival in this life.

Let me give you a very simple and basic example. The cat's instinct and intellect make her run after the mouse for food or run after any type of meat. The cat's intellect makes her pick up her kitten with her teeth without hurting it and take it to a safer place when her instinct tells her there is a danger surrounding her kitten. A cat will pick her kitten up by the neck using her teeth, without causing it any harm. The cat's intellect compels the cat to go out of sight when she wants to defecate, just as the cat's intellect compels her to bury her waste upon finishing her defecation. These actions don't happen accidentally; meaning the animal's intellect is connected to the anatomical aspect. The animal has a connection between the way that they are made and their surrounding environment and how they are born and how they live.

The human intellect is different because the human has the mental capacity to invent new things like the car or a computer. The human intellect can initiate and has the free will to choose and to learn. With the human, there is always room for development and progress, mentally and intellectually. This process starts with sperm and ova until the last day of life. Always there is room for progress and development. Especially in the first stage of our life. That explains why the first years of any baby's life are the most important years to learn new things, like walking, running, reading, writing, and talking. The reason for this is there is a huge number of synapses and brain cells that are growing and developing at a very fast rate. Animals learn by instinct when they look at their surrounding environment that they are born into. Humans learn by the intellect, by memorization, repetition, learning, and experience.

There is a difference between the animal and the plant to us as human beings, for a variety of reasons which are:

1. We have more interaction and stronger bonds with animals than with plants because we think that plants are less active than animals, for this reason, we have less interaction with plants

2. We might have the plant for beauty, to make us feel calm and give us a nice environment, like flowers in the garden, or a garden of green grass or any beautiful scene. Plants are not designed to live with us especially for a long period, e.g., if you pick a flower from the garden and you bring it into your home, the flower will not survive as it has been removed from the environment in which it is designed to

live. As I said earlier, the world is built on the Yin and Yang and the five elements. Now the flower is deprived of five important things for its existence, 1. earth, 2. air, 3. water, 4. sun, 5. carbon dioxide.

3. When we buy our food to eat, we think only about filling our hunger, we do not keep the food to interact with it. For this reason, the food will not last as long with us for interaction or bond. But with the animal, the story is completely different and our interaction and bond might last all our lives for the following reasons:

   a) Animals have a certain amount of intellect in addition to their Instinct which they are born with.
   b) You could see your cat giving birth to her new-born kittens. You are interacting with them from the first moment they come to this life, so with time, these kittens know you are their owner because of the interaction, the bond, the care, and attention they are getting from you and this applies to every other pet or animal.
   c) Humans establish a mutual emotional relationship with their animals and vice versa. That explains why the owner misses their pet and the pet misses them because animals know who is their owner and they know when they come or they leave, and they know if their owner is sick or worried, this is related to the universal karma, this is related to the oneness and the interaction of all the universe as one unit.

Later I will talk about it in more detail when I talk about karma from an Oriental perspective, now let me give you a very simple example from personal experience.

One day when I was lecturing and saying how from an Oriental perspective that every organ is connected to a certain tissue in the human body and this tissue is linked to the emotional state that this person is feeling. At the same time, I said, for example, lungs are related to sadness and grief and the tissue they control is the skin and they control the hair of the body, except for the hair of the head which is controlled by the kidney from an Oriental perspective. That also explains why when we have asthma, we can have eczema and psoriasis with it.

One of the students said to me, that is amazing because when her mother died her cat's hair fell out almost completely. When she took the cat to the vet, he said to her that this is due to the recent shock and very sad news which made the skin change and the hair fall out. The cat or any other animal knows when their owner is sick and when the owner is worried and they know when their owner dies. They cannot express themselves verbally and even if they can do so we cannot understand them, but they start to show remarkable signs, like not coming back to the house or being very quiet or less active, and in some cases, they stop eating completely and lose weight.

No one can measure the sadness and the grief of the animal when their owner dies or conversely the sadness and the grief the owner will have when their pet dies. We do know from an Oriental perspective and human instinct that if you have a bond with your pet, and the more interaction you will have with them the deeper the grief and sadness will be and vice versa. Many, still remember their first-ever pet and indeed they might not be able to forget them for the rest of their lives.

The list of the Yin and Yang is endless, all what I have spoken about in the previous chapters about the Yin and Yang is from a tangible, material, visible and substantial aspect, and perspective.

"It is better to teach or live equality and love ... than to have hatred and prejudice."

Rosa Parks

That concludes the refresher/introduction
part to Oriental Medicine.

PART 4

THE FUNCTIONS OF THE FIVE ELEMENTS

CHAPTER 1

THE FUNCTION OF THE LUNGS

(1) The lungs open into the nose
(2) Produces the voice and controls the Qi
(3) Controls hair on the body and Skin
(4) Descending and Dispersing
(5) Controls Water Passage
(6) Channels and Blood Vessels
(7) Sadness and Grief

From a western perspective, the lungs have one function and that is inhalation and exhalation. Taking in Oxygen and expelling Carbon Dioxide. As we mentioned earlier, the yin organ has a yang job to do, Yang is movement and activity, no rest. From an oriental perspective the lungs have 6 functions:

1. The lungs open into the nose

You breathe through your nose. If you breathe through your mouth you will damage the kidneys and bladder and you will wake up with a salty taste in your mouth (the function of kidneys is to regulate salt/potassium). When exercising you breathe through the mouth to get rid of CO_2 faster so that you don't become fatigued. If you don't get rid of the CO_2 build-up, Urea, and Lactic acid build-up so you will get spasms and cramps.

When you are exercising you should breathe normally, but out through the mouth. In the nose you have very tiny hairs, their job is to purify and filter the oxygen and air to prevent viruses, bacteria and germs from entering the lungs and respiratory system. Also, the function of the nose is to warm up the air, to create a balance between the internal and external environment. If you breathe through your mouth the air is not being purified. It goes straight to the tonsils – the first gate in the immune, respiratory system and lymph system. If you are sick you lose your sense of smell – the immune system is affected. The Sinus connects the nose to the facial cavity. If your sinus is blocked everything will be blocked. Then you're creating an environment for Bacteria and Virus – flu and infection because of stagnation.

If you have your tonsils taken out you are susceptible to flu, colds, and infections. As we are talking now there are millions of germs, bacteria, viruses, in the air. We cannot stop ourselves from inhaling them. They will be part of our breathing. In this case, the immune system, lymphatic system, respiratory system, endocrine system are on emergency call 24 hours to prevent the pathogenic invaders like the germs, bacteria, virus entering the body. In the first stage of a cold, the immune system engages in a battle with the help of the lymphatic system with germs, bacteria, and viruses. This battle takes place in the upper respiratory tract – nose, sinus, tonsils, If the immune system is strong you will be able to defeat the pathogenic invaders. This means you will only have cold symptoms:

1. Very slight temperature
2. Runny nose – mostly white fluids
3. Runny eyes – every cavity tries to expel it
4. Muscle pain, weakness, stiffness

5. Slight tiredness
6. Slight pale complexion

All these symptoms will disappear without intervention. In this case, your immune system has won the battle, and these symptoms will disappear. If your immune system is weak the pathogenic Invaders will win the battle and now, they will go farther down. It will be your lower respiratory tract which consists of the trachea, bronchi, bronchioles, lungs, diaphragm and pleura cavity (fluid). You will have symptoms of flu:

1. Yellow/Green sputum mucus from the nose
2. Body temperature getting higher
3. Start to sweat more and more
4. Body shivering to preserve heat
5. More tired – no energy
6. Symptoms of cold worsened
7. Very pale

This then progresses to a chest infection. Then invades the fluid in the lungs – chest will rattle. Both cold and flu can be either bacterial or viral. Bacteria is yang. It is active, fire. Viral is yin. It is rest, water. Bacteria attacks quickly (yang) and when you attack it with antibiotics it will die quickly. Antibiotics won't kill the virus because it is dormant and could be there since the womb.

There are millions of viruses in the body, you can't live without them. The liver, lymphatic system, the immune system attacks the germs like a laser when they enter the body (e.g. from your hands). If your tonsils are gone, the germs enter down and turn to flu. The first gate is gone. In the stage of a cold, to help the immune system take the natural antibiotic (orange, ½ apple, black pepper, a spoon of honey, lemon juice, vinegar, garlic, onion). Take this as many times a day as you like, as a juice or paste, however not on an empty stomach. Also, drink vinegar and lemon juice – not water – all the time. This cannot be taken on an empty stomach. Take at least 2 fingers of vinegar. When you go to the bathroom you wash your hands, take a shower and use shampoo and soap. You are washing your body from the outside. The natural antibiotic and the vinegar and lemon juice wash the body from the inside like an internal shampoo and will help the liver and immune system to detoxify.

2. Produces the voice and controls the Qi

The power of the voice depends on the strength of your lungs primarily and all your respiratory system in general. Strong lung qi gives the person a very strong and powerful voice and vice-versa. The qi forces the voice out, Example – people with Asthma have a weak voice. The power of the voice depends on the interaction between the vocal cord and the lung's atmospheric pressure (the hydraulic pressure). If you have a weak lung qi there will be no descending and you will have constipation. There is not enough power for defecation.

3. Controls hair on the body and Skin

The lungs from an oriental perspective represent the endocrine system, lymphatic system and respiratory system. The endocrine system is related to hormones. The treatment principle here is to check the gland affected (it is mostly the thyroid) and treat the hormone. If there is too much Testosterone treat the lungs and kidneys. While you are sitting your heart rate is between 70-80 beats a minute. What will happen when you start running? Running is a physical and muscular activity. It requires oxygen and fuel. This fuel needs to be supplied to the working muscles, in this case to all your body specifically your arms and legs. Your lungs start to take more oxygen. Your heart will take the oxygen, pumped up by the lungs, to the bloodstream. It will be carried with the heart circulation to the working muscles. At the same time, the liver releases Glycogen as a form of Glucose to supply the nutrients and the fluids required to the working muscles to sustain the action. This process produces waste. After a while, your body produces chemical toxins. Your body will be able to get rid of some of them and will not be able to get rid of others. The skin is the biggest organ in the human body that helps the excretion of the toxins through the process of sweating.

To look at it differently generally speaking in most cases we might have asthma, psoriasis, eczema, dermatitis, we have skin problems with it. Acne can be hormonal and may be related to the lungs however Acne can be related to other organs. The skin is the uppermost external environment in the human body. It is the first thing that meets the external environment. The skin is the mediator between the internal and external environments. It is part of the immune system. Why? It protects against pathogenic invaders entering the body. If you are sick you start to sweat. This is a form of protection. When you are sick your temperature goes high and you start sweating through the skin. This is a form of protection to maintain the temperature at the right level. A message goes from the brain to the Hypothalamus (human thermostat) to say the temperature is getting higher. The skin capillaries dilate and open the pores for the body to release the toxins. When you run you sweat, the brain sends a message and the capillaries start to dilate. When you stop running (you are in rest) it's the opposite process. Your body no longer needs the same amount of oxygen, the heart doesn't need to pump as fast, and the liver doesn't need to supply Glycogen. The parasympathetic is taking place (to slow). When your breath is back to normal and the heart rate is at a normal level, the temperature drops and the sweating stops. A message goes from the brain to the hair follicles and skin capillaries close. If you stop doing the activity and the heart keeps beating fast and the lungs are still breathing fast and you are still sweating this is a sign of trouble. The sweat should evaporate when you stop. When you are sick, white blood cells go up to fight the infection. A message is sent from the brain to the immune system to tell them to multiply.

White Blood Cells = yang – they go up to fight the infection.

Red Blood Cells = Yin.

When you get well the message goes from the brain to the immune system to stop producing white blood cells. Red blood cells go back up = you look well and rosy. Red Blood cells carry oxygen. White Blood cells carry antibodies. Generally speaking, if the immune system doesn't respond to the message of the brain and continues to white blood, this results in two cases:

a) You will still have an infection

b) If the person is healthy and the white blood cells continue, this means the body is entering into cancerous cells – means Leukaemia (blood cancer). The white blood cells have taken over and are working against the body.

There are different reasons why the immune system wouldn't respond: injury to the brain or too many antibiotics. The Brain is not fixed in the head, it moves like swimming in a pool. That's why when you stand up quickly you feel dizzy. The older you get the more the brain shrinks. This leaves more space for crap. Work on the head and neck to rejuvenate the oxygen. Massage the head and squeeze the neck.

4. Descending and Dispersing

Descending means sending something down, the lungs need to descend the air and oxygen that we inhale. They descend this air and oxygen to all body organs and systems and every part of our body, from the hair on top of the head to the sole of feet. Without oxygen, our body, cells, and organs would not be able to survive. From a western perspective dispersing represents diffusion. This is a process of spreading out the oxygen and the body fluids to the skin. As we said earlier, the lungs control the hair on the body and the skin, the skin is the biggest organ in the human body, it is the organ that links and connects the external environment with the internal environment.

Air qi is Yang qi. Blood is Yin qi: The lungs are responsible for the descending and dispersing of any form of qi to all body parts. For example, the lungs descend the air qi, mixing it with the blood and pushing blood qi, yin qi, yang qi, lymph qi, and fluid qi. The stronger your breath is the stronger the qi is to push circulation and qi and to get everything moving.

5. Controls Water Passage (Skin Pores)

As we said earlier the lungs are connected to the skin as a tissue. The skin holds the pores. These pores are responsible for regulating body temperature through the process of sweating and evaporation. When you run you need oxygen. Oxygen (air qi) and food (food qi) come together to produce the energy that you require to do your action. The outcome of the action is the production of lactic acid and urea and the build-up of waste. All these come together to form the sweat. The skin pores have to open and the hair on the skin allows the sweat to leave the body and to regulate the body temperature to prevent heat stroke from occurring. If the build-up of toxins in the body continues over a long period in addition to the exercise this will eventually lead to multiple organ failure. For example, drinking excessive alcohol will lead to cirrhosis of the liver; one of the most important functions of the liver is to continuously detoxify the body. The best way to describe the liver from an oriental perspective is like an internal washing machine, continuously washing your body even while you are asleep. What will happen to the kidney if we don't allow sweat to leave the body? The communication between the kidney and lungs is very important as both of them share the same two processes. Process one is breathing, process two is expelling body fluid.

The lungs with the help of the skin get rid of sweat as a fluid and the kidney with the help of the urinary bladder gets rid of the fluid as a form of urine. In process one both the lung and the kidney are responsible for the respiratory process. This explains why from an oriental perspective there are two types of Asthma, yin Asthma and yang Asthma. If you have difficulty breathing in during the inhalation process this is called a yin Asthma which is related to your kidney as an organ. In this case, the kidney is not gripping the air qi. As an emotion this Asthma is related to fear itself, panic attack, being nervous and to any form of shock. Whether it is emotional, physical, and mental or any type of shock, they will all interfere with the breathing process, particularly inhalation.

If you are not able to breathe out in the exhalation this is called yang asthma which is related to your lungs as an organ. The lungs do not have the power or strength to push open the airway, sinus, nose and/or mouth to let the air out. This is caused by weak lung qi. The emotional aspect linked to the exhalation and the lungs is sadness, grief, and negative complaining. The exhalation process holds the aspect of letting go especially emotions.

If your Asthma or Eczema is caused by sadness or grief the cream or inhaler that the doctor gives you will give you relief and might ease your symptoms however they are not designed to solve your emotional problems. In this case, the cream or inhaler is dealing with the manifestation; they are not dealing with the root cause. This is the difference between oriental medicine and western clinical medicine. Six people might come to the clinic with Asthma, this means the title of their complaint is the same however when we check the tongue and the pulse, we find that the root cause of each client's condition is different from one another. For example, Asthma might be caused by sadness and grief, or by anger or by heavy periods and anxiety. The list is endless. This is applied to any medical condition from an oriental perspective whether the condition is physical, emotional or mental. When all of these emotions and toxins are not being released for long periods, they will eventually lead to kidney failure. The kidney fails in expelling the urine due to the huge amount of toxin which is built up and the reason for it, in this case, is when the sweating process is interrupted.

6. Channels and Blood Vessels

As we said earlier, we have twelve channels, six in each arm which are replicated and also six in each foot, also replicated. Channels are a line of energy through which the qi flows continuously. Qi can't flow without breathing. This means the air qi from lungs pushes the blood qi in the vessels, these vessels are a network of veins, which are a muscular tube and carry oxygen. As vessels spread through the body, they form tiny hair-like vessels, these are smaller in size and shape and are called capillaries. The capillaries and our nerve endings reach every part of our body. This is part of the diffusion process. This means the lungs have to diffuse the blood, oxygen and nutrients to every part in our body. This means air qi is yang and blood qi is yin. Qi pushes blood, blood nourishes qi.

The interaction between blood and qi will lead to the production of the pulse. The pulse is defined as a life force, if you have no pulse there is no life. The power and strength of the pulse depend on your circulation. Your circulation also depends on many factors for example; if you have a lot of cholesterol it will lead to a blockage in your vessels which makes the hearts job harder to pump through a narrow vein or artery. In this case, your pulse might be strong, and this is an indication and a sign of high blood pressure. The best way to describe high blood pressure and compare it to low blood pressure is o compare it to a car tyre, one tyre is full of air and ready to explode, representing high blood pressure, this tyre will need to be deflated to allow some of the pressure out, another tyre being flat representing low blood pressure, this tyre will need more air put into it to keep it at a certain standard level. In addition to these twelve channels, we have two other channels, the front is called the Ren and is connected to all our body organs, the back is called the Du and is connected to our nerve system and spinal cord. Each spinal cord is linked through the brain into an organ and through the spine into emotions. The urinary bladder channel is the largest in the human body, it starts from the corner of the eye and circulates twice around the spine, and ends on the little toe. The point on the spine measuring 1.5 cun from the spine represents your emotional aspect. Also from an oriental perspective, the spine represents your immune system and lymphatic system.

7. Sadness and Grief

The emotional aspect connected to the lungs is sadness and grief. As we said earlier, there are a lot of things in life that can make us sad. We cannot be constantly happy, and we cannot be constantly sad. We try our best to find the perfect, but it is not always easy to do. Some people can cope with situations better than others however generally speaking when we talk 93% of our conversation is related to the past. We rarely speak about the present. This means dwelling on the past is like a chicken sitting on an egg, incubating it. Most of our sadness and grief comes from our past and we drag it into our future.

When sadness and grief are combined with anger, hatred, resentment, frustration and jealousy this combination is disastrous. In some cases, it can turn a normal person into a person with psychiatric and mental issues. It is not fair to say to a person 'don't get sad' or 'don't worry'. At the end of the day, we are all human, we are not stone. We should get sad if the situation for it arises, however, don't hold on to it but instead let it go. However, the problem is that for some people when they are sad they want everybody around them to be sad and feel the way they're feeling. This is part of their selfish ego. Sadness and grief for a long period will be like a burden sitting on your chest. It will prevent you from breathing. Crying is a form of healing and purification and it also holds the aspect of letting go.

The Liver opens into the eyes and the liver holds the aspect of anger, hatred, resentment and frustration. When we cry our tears come through the eyes. If you don't cry to let go the sadness and grief will sit on top of the chest. This will build up and will form a qi stagnation and aggregation. This qi will be like a lump in the throat and this emotional lump for a long period will lead to a physical lump and will trigger the start of cancer anywhere in the body but specifically in the throat, lungs or breast and especially the left breast because of its location over the heart as the heart carries out emotional state.

From an oriental perspective there are four types of crying:

1. Happy – this is related to your heart as an organ and also the pericardium (muscular sac around the heart). It is also related to the heart a. pericardium as channels because the heart is related to excitement, joy and happiness. This explains why some people will drop dead when they hear happy news.

2. Sad – this is related to your lungs. The lungs are related to sadness and grief. It will be a lot worse if you are sad and physically you are unable to cry. Sometimes people will drop dead when they hear sudden news; this depends on their

emotional state and where they are at the time when they hear the news.

3. The third type of crying is not related to being happy or sad. It is triggered by the use of a certain combination of needles to open all the water passages to make the aspect of letting go and to make the person attach deeply to their emotional feelings. Imagine the person as a layer of onion and the emotion is embedded in this onion. You need to go deep down to the layer which holds the emotional feeling. We need to find what chakra is blocked and where the emotions are held and what channels or organs are affected.

4. Infants cry as a form of communication.

Generally speaking, the chakra is deeply affected by our emotional feelings. The reason for this is every chakra is related to an organ and related to a nerve plexus which connects to our emotions. Another reason is that the chakra is restricted and is in a smaller place than the channel. It might take a longer time for the channel to be blocked but it takes very little time for the chakra to be blocked.

Sometimes crying can be related to your hormonal state which also plays a major part in the chakra system and in the way that you feel. For example, from a female aspect, you might cry before, during, or after ovulation, and also pregnant woman might find that their emotions fluctuate from crying to laughing, from being normal to being depressed. The emotions and hormones have a major impact on all our body functions especially digestion. This explains why a pregnant woman will love a certain food during a certain time of her pregnancy and the next day they can't tolerate the same food.

Generally speaking, breathing is the first process and is the aspect that will be affected by our emotional state and the way we feel. Every process and every function will be affected by our breathing. For example, when you worry your breathing is impaired, now the digestive system will start to pay the price and the stomach as an organ will start to pay the price. Why? Because when you are worried you lose your appetite, or you are unable to taste food in your mouth. This is an example of the effect and impact of the emotional state on your body's physical function. In this case the digestive as a system and the stomach as an organ.

The Lungs form a Five Element Perspective

> *Element – Metal*

The Lungs represent the metal aspect from a five-element perspective. The Lungs also represent the metal spect as a taste, for example, if you are sick with a cold or flu you will have a metal taste in your mouth, sometimes people describe it as being like a taste of blood. The reason for the metal taste in the mouth is because if there is an excess of mucus, damp or phlegm, all of these fluids will fill the lungs. As we said earlier, the Lungs open into the nose and the sinus cavity. The excess fluids will go up into the nose and will block the nose and the sinus completely. Over a long period, this will descend to the stomach, resulting in indigestion and a loss of sense of taste. In some cases, the build-up of fluids in the nose and sinus can result in bad breath.

As we mentioned earlier, the Lungs are Yin and the Large Intestine is Yang. If the Lungs are affected your bowel movement will also be affected. For example, if you have asthma this means you have a weak lung qi and weak bowel movement and constipation. This is because the defecation process is affected. Another example is when the lungs and sinus are blocked due to cold invasion you will have a white discharge through the nose and also a white mucus discharge through the bowel. People with Crohn's disease or Ulcerative Colitis will have a white mucus discharge if they drink a lot of cold drinks however if they drink alcohol or eat hot spicy food the discharge will be yellow or brown and also with mucus. The white discharge is caused by excess cold in the body which leads to Yang deficiency. Yang has the function of warming and to push up.

> *Direction – East and Right*

The Lungs represent the west and left as a direction. From an anatomy and physiology perspective, the right lung is bigger than the left because of the location of the heart. The west represents the moon and is related to night-time. The Liver represents east and right as a direction. The east represents the sun and so is related to daytime. The east is where the sun rises and so is related to heat. If you have a cough caused by excess heat the cough will be worse in the daytime. If you have a cough caused by excess cold the cough will be worse in the night-time. If the cough is related to yin deficiency the cooling and moistening aspect of the lungs is being decreased and diminished. With a cough due to yin deficiency the cough could be at any time of the day however it will be particularly worse at night, the cough will also be dry and may be accompanied by sweating from the palms of the hands, armpits, chest, breast area and back of the neck.

The difference between a dry cough and a wet cough is that the dry cough does not produce mucus and will be tickly. The heat from this type of cough may travel down to the sole of the feet and the urine will be very yellow and dark with a strong smell. This is what creates the relationship between the Lungs and Kidneys both from anatomy and physiology point of view and also from an oriental point of view. If you have difficulty breathing in this form of asthma is related to the Kidney's (functions of the Kidneys is to grip and hold the qi). If you have difficulty breathing out this is yang asthma and is related to the Lungs not being able to finish the exhalation process.

> ### *Stage of Life – Young Adult*

The Lungs represent the stage of life known as a 'young adult'. This is the part of your life after you have passed through the baby and adolescence stage and where you want to establish your career and start to think of starting your own family.

> ### *Season – Autumn*

The Lungs represent autumn as a season. The autumn is the time of year, when the leaves start to fall from the trees. The same can be applied to human life when the hair starts to fall out and turns grey. It is a physical, emotional and transitional stage of life. At this time of our life, we start to have more sense and logic and we start to slow down in our processes in life.

NOTES

_____

_____

_____

_____

_____

_____

_____

_____

_____

_____

_____

_____

"Our Greatest Glory Is Not In Never Falling,
But In Rising Every Time We Fall."
Nelson Mandela

CHAPTER 2

PATTERNS OF THE LUNGS

The lungs are the two organs that belong to the respiratory system. They are two muscular sacs that are filled with fluid which is yin in nature and has the function of cooling and moistening. The function of the lungs fluid from a western perspective is to prevent friction between the lungs and the surrounding structures such as the ribs and diaphragm during breathing. The respiratory system consists of two parts, the upper respiratory tract, and the lower respiratory tract. The upper respiratory tract consists of the following: Nose, Sinus, Throat, and the Tonsils. The lower respiratory tract consists of Trachea Bronchi, Bronchiole, Alveoli, Lungs, Pleura Cavity, Diaphragm, Ribs, and intercostal muscles.

The function of the lungs from a western perspective is to take the oxygen from the outside environment and send it to the heart to be circulated all of the body's tissues and organs down to the cellular level. There are two phases involved in the process of taking in the oxygen by the lungs and descending it and dispersing it through the circulation of the heart and the blood to all of our body, these processes are called inhalation and exhalation.

The process of inhalation is the process of breathing in oxygen. The diaphragm is a muscular wall and can relax and contract. When we breathe in the diaphragm becomes flat in a horizontal way and pulls up the two lungs and the two sides of the ribs down. This action increases the lung's shape and size and allows the air to rush in. The action is helped by the diaphragm and the intercostal muscles and from a western perspective is called inhalation. From an oriental perspective, the inhalation process depends on the strength and the power of your kidney qi especially kidney yang.

When we breathe out the opposite takes place, the diaphragm becomes dome-shaped pointing upwards and decreases the size and shape of the lungs to squeeze the air and carbon dioxide out to the upper respiratory tract. This is called exhalation from a western perspective. The breathing out, from an oriental perspective, depends on the power and strength of our lungs to clear and expel the ai rout of the internal environment.

Lung Qi Deficiency

This condition is caused by the invasion of the lungs by any form of wind. From an oriental, there are two types of asthma., yin asthma and yang asthma. If you have asthma and you have difficulty breathing in this is regarded as yin asthma because when we breathe in the air has to go down and as we said the yin descended. This yin asthma is caused by a weakness in our kidneys. As we know, one of the functions of the yang is to warm and push up. If there is lung qi deficiency and kidney yang deficiency this will lead to difficulty breathing especially in the inhalation and will also lead to frequent urination. Frequent urination occurs because the lungs descend the fluid down, a process which is equivalent to diffusion from a western perspective, the kidneys do not have enough qi or yang to hold the fluid and grip the qi hence the person will have frequent urination sometimes lead to dryness with a salty taste in the mouth.

Yang Asthma (When the lungs are not able to exhale)

When a person has difficulty breathing it could be due to a variety of reasons. The weakness in the lungs from an anatomy and physiology perspective leads to lung qi deficiency. Any obstruction to the airway whether to the sinus, the windpipe, or the lungs by phlegm, mucus, damp or fluid will lead to lung qi deficiency and will affect our breathing process. It will also affect the functional aspect of diffusion of the lungs which is descending and dispersing from an oriental perspective and diffusion from a western perspective. Our sinus is the first gate in our respiratory system and if they are blocked our respiratory, immune, and lymphatic systems will pay the price. The blockage of the sinus will create an environment for infection and inflammation because bacteria want a damp, dark, and stagnated environment. People who have blocked sinus for a long period will get a lot of sinus infections and ear infections because the immune and lymphatic systems are not being activated due to the stagnation.

From an oriental perspective if you have difficulty breathing in this is related to your kidneys and our nervous system because the kidneys control shock and represent the state of being nervous and panicking and being fearful. If you have difficulty breathing out this is related to sadness and grief and from an anatomy and physiology perspective, it is related to your respiratory as a system, your skin as a system, and to your lungs as an organ. Also, if there is anger, hatred, jealousy, resentment, or frustration the qi will be stagnant in the chest and upper Jiao area and any structure in the same area will be affected. This explains why women will have tender breasts, especially the left breast, because the heart captures the mind and the pericardium carries all of our emotions, and the left breast is located near to the heart and pericardium.

The lungs are related to sadness and grief and the heart is related to joy and excitement and there will be emotional conflict. This conflict is represented by the lungs on one side because they try to descend the qi downwards and the liver on the other side because it obstructs the qi from descending causing it to stagnate. There are a variety of reasons which cause the lung qi to stagnate such as too much phlegm, dampness, carbon dioxide, or postural and structural issues related to your anatomy and physiology. Regardless of what the root cause is our job is to create the perfect balance from every aspect whether psychological, structural, physical, sexual, or emotional.

Wind-Cold Invading the Lungs

When wind-cold starts to invade the lungs, the person will have the following symptoms:

- Itchy, tickly throat
- Blocked nose and sinus
- White watery mucus discharge
- Tongue – white coating
- Pulse – weak and empty, especially on the lung pulse

From a western perspective, all of the symptoms above are an indication that the person has an ordinary cold. The reason why the person has each of the symptoms is detailed below. Itchy, tickly throat When the bacteria or germ attacks our body they attack it suddenly and abruptly.

From an oriental perspective, our muscular system and our skin are a big part of our immune system and they form a barrier which makes the Wei qi (immune system) and the muscles strong and to contract, and the skin pores to close to preserve heat and to stop the bacteria and the germ from entering inside our body.

From a western perspective, the same process as above takes place but at a different location. When our body is being attacked the bacteria and germ enter our immune and lymphatic systems, if they are strong in general, will stop the bacteria and germ from descending into our respiratory tracts. This means our immune system and our lymphatic system engage in a battle with the bacteria and germ and this battle takes place inside the throat where our tonsils and lymphatic glands are located on the sides of the neck, hence why the person will have an itchy and tickly throat. Our tonsils and lymphatic glands form the first defense line in the face of pathogenic invaders whether it is a germ or a bacteria. If the persons' tonsils have been taken out they will be more susceptible to cold and flu because their first defensive line is gone which makes it easier for bacteria and germs to descend downwards to our lungs and our lower respiratory system. If the persons immune and lymphatic systems are strong and the person is not under any form of stress then these systems will be able to defeat the bacteria and germ and prevent them from descending into the lungs hence the cold will run it's course without any form of treatment whether oriental or western.

Blocked Nose and Sinus and White Watery Discharge

The battle that takes place between the pathogenic invaders and the immune and lymphatic systems takes place in the upper respiratory tract, the nose and sinus will become blocked and at the start, the nose will become runny with a clear nasal discharge. This is because the glands in our neck are working as hard as possible to prevent the germ or bacteria from going down to our lower respiratory tract. If our immune system loses the battle then our nose and sinus will become blocked and obstructed with the white sticky mucus discharge and this discharge becomes stagnant and is no longer runny. The person will start to develop a slight temperature and will feel a little bit weak and lethargic with headaches and muscle pain. Generally speaking, this is just an ordinary cold that will not have as much impact on our health in general.

CHAPTER 3

THE FUNCTION OF THE LIVER

From a western perspective, the Liver is a very important organ in the human body and has multiple functions. The following is a brief description of the functions of the Liver and its corresponding organ the Gallbladder. The liver produces a lot of enzymes that work by creating a chemical reaction to assist the body function. One of the most important functions of the liver is to wash the body internally. From an oriental perspective, this is best described as being similar to a washing machine. The Liver washes and detoxifies the body whether you are awake or asleep, active, or at rest.

The paired organ with the liver is the Gallbladder. The Gallbladder is a yang organ with a yin job to do. The function of the Gallbladder is to store bile. Bile helps your digestive system break down fats.

The Liver is a yin organ and has a yang job to do which is the metabolism, meaning the action of burning releasing energy.

The bile is a form of fluid. The fluid is yin however the function of the bile is yang. The function of the bile is to burn body fat, burning means heat and heat is yang. This explains why if a person has their Gallbladder removed by surgery, regardless of the reason for it, this means the aspect of burning and metabolizing the fat in the body is either gone completely or massively decreased. Also, if a person eats a dry form of food especially fatty, oily, greasy, and hot or spicy food they will have the following: indigestion, belching, and heartburn. They may also occasionally have trapped wind which leads to excess flatulence or excess hiccupping. Why? Because the wind has to pass, whether it passes through the mouth or the back passage. If the wind is not passed it will either rise and obstruct the chest resulting in difficult and heavy breathing especially with the exhalation, or it will descend down and as it is not being released it will create a huge form or pressure and discomfort and often accompanied by a very sharp and intense pain that the person finds it difficult to cope with. If a person has gallstones the pain will be very sharp and severe and sometimes can be so severe that the pain travels up to the back where the scapula is. This is where one of the points of the small intestine is.

From an oriental perspective, if the Gallbladder is removed, then from a functional aspect the Lungs will take over. How? Because when you do physical activity the body needs two types of fuel, it will need oxygen which is taken by the Lungs from the external environment and it will Glycogen which is released by the Liver as a form of Glucose. The body will also need the function of the Heart which is circulating both the Oxygen and the Glycogen to the working muscles to sustain the action. All of these processes are yang in nature, and they will compensate for the Gallbladder which has been removed, you may still have indigestion and heartburn, especially if you eat late at night. Daytime is yang, night-time is yin and the gastric juices in the Stomach are yin because they are a form of juice and fluid however their function in the body is yang, to aid digestion. This means that movement and activity after eating will help the digestion and excretion and will help in burning the body fat and by doing so will help to relieve all the symptoms we mentioned earlier.

The Liver and Gallbladder need to function in harmony to function to their optimum and maximum health. For example, drinking alcohol will damage the liver; if the Liver is damaged automatically the Gallbladder will pay the price for this damage, and vice versa if there is a blockage in the bile duct, the Liver will pay the price for it. The eyes are an indication of this, one of the Liver's functions is that it opens into the eyes if the Gallbladder is blocked the eyes will be yellow. Eventually, over a long period, this will spread all over your body and will manifest and show itself on your skin as a yellow complexion as with Jaundice and Hepatitis. The reason for the manifestation in the skin is because the liver and skin both play a major role in detoxifying the body. The Liver washes the body internally to expel the toxins and build up from any internal process whether it's from digestion, excretion, or so on. The skin is the largest organ in the human body and acts as a mediator and a protector between the internal and external environment. The skin and the Liver are booth part of the immune system. Both the skin and the liver have the job of keeping the body pure and clean and detoxified. The skin does this through the process of sweating. This explains why if the bile is building up it will go to the highest level or to the highest organ in the human body which is the skin and so not only will the eyes appear yellow but the skin also will appear yellow.

If we want to link the Liver to the Lungs – the lungs control the skin and the hair on the body. If the skin is yellow due to a dysfunction of the liver, the physical activity you do will help release the toxin throughout the sweat. In this case, it will be decreased through the sweating process. Another form of excretion is through urination. Drinking a lot of water, especially water that doesn't contain Fluoride, will help the excretion through the Kidneys and is another form of helping the Liver and the Gallbladder.

From an oriental perspective the Liver has six functions in the human body:

1. Ensures the smooth flow of qi
2. Stores blood
3. Manifests in the nails
4. Controls Sinews (Ligament, Cartilage, Tendon, Tissue)
5. Opens into the eyes
6. Controls the ethereal soul

1. Ensures the smooth flow of qi

If Liver Qi flows freely and smoothly all of the qi in our body systems and organs will flow smoothly and freely. This then means that all other systems and organs will function to their optimum level of health and well-being. From a five-element point of view, the Liver represents the baby stage of life. Why is this? Because the liver represents the spark and the start of human life which determines the other stages in our life. For example, when you sit in your car and turn on the ignition this is the spark that will determine every other process which takes place in the car's function. If the car doesn't start then the other processes will not take place such as fuel consumption, water circulation, and the battery will not start. These processes all depend on the first action and the first stage of the car function which is turning it on at the ignition. The Liver represents the spark that is similar to the ignition in the car.

The Liver ensures the smooth flow of qi according to the following:

1) Your physical activity
2) Your time of the month
3) Whether you are male or female

When we talk about females specifically, we mean the time of the ovulation and the time of the period. Later I will explain why, from an oriental perspective, women will sometimes have heavy, irregular, scanty, short or long periods or bleeding between periods and identify which organ is affected and what emotions are influencing the time of the period and the time of ovulation.

Physical Activity

When you are not doing any physical activity, which requires cardiovascular action your heart will beat between 70 and 80 beats a minute. When you start to run or jog these are the physical activities and they require oxygen, blood, and glucose as a form of energy, three organs have to come together to sustain the physical action that requires fuel:

a) You start to breathe fast; the Lungs will increase the air intake to supply to the working muscles

b) The Heart is the muscle at the centre of the circulatory system pumping blood around your body as it beats. This blood delivers oxygen and nutrients to all parts of the body, and carries away unwanted carbon dioxide and waste products.

c)   The Liver as an organ has to release the energy which is store as a form of Glycogen in the Liver to be released as a form of Glucose. This is why Glucose drinks are taken by sportsmen and women.

The Liver releases the Glycogen as a form of Glucose, which is a form of fluid and sugar, with the help of the Pancreas. If two people do the same type of exercise and one of them eats two burgers before the exercise and the other drinks a sweet drink then the person who takes the drink will perform better and will release energy faster to the working muscles. The person who ate the burgers will not perform as well because the burgers will have to pass through each stage that the digestion process requires from chewing the food to allowing it to go down to the Stomach for the Stomach to produce the gastric enzymes and juices for the digestion, to sending it down to the small intestine which is where most of our absorption takes place before it turns the remainder to waste and sends it down to the large intestine. All of these processes take a long time to release the energy required to the working muscles. Also, because the final process will be the elimination of waste as a form of stool, this means that at the time of physical activity the body is dealing with the toxin also. The blood is going to the digestion and the bowel in addition to the working muscles and therefore the performance will not be to its optimum level.

The difference between the two is that when you have just had the sweet drink the body does not need to pass through the stages I mentioned earlier and the glucose will be released through the Liver immediately to the working muscles. Prophet Muhammad PBUH gave a very good health prescription 'before you eat, think about three things – your Stomach is divided into three parts, one third is for your food, another third for your water intake and the last third is for air intake breathing'. When you overeat, you are not leaving enough space for the air. The same could be applied to eating before bedtime. It is not good to eat less than three hours before bedtime. The reason for this is that your brain is responsible for your physical activity and physical processes in addition to digestion. The brain is responsible for your conscious stage and is related to your sympathetic nerve system, which speeds things up from a western perspective. From an oriental perspective, the sympathetic nerve system represents yang as Yang speeds things up. When you go to bed to sleep your parasympathetic system along with your subconscious and your mind have to take over the process. This is because the sleeping process is a non-physical, non-tangible, non-substantial process. Sleeping is not related to your physical body and it is not connected to any structural organ. Sleeping is connected to your subconscious and your mind and also to your emotional state. When you eat or drink the food and drink goes downward. When you breathe, the air goes downwards. The blood has to go down to the Stomach to the digestive system to start the digestive process. At the same time, the brain needs enough oxygen and glucose to pass through the four stages of sleep. In this case, the person is creating a large conflict between the brain (which is responsible for the physical aspect of digestion) and the subconscious and the mind (which are responsible for the sleeping process). Instead of ascending to the brain, the oxygen and glucose descend to the Stomach. This explains why the person will either not be able to fall asleep in the first place or they will not be able to have a peaceful night's sleep. They may also have difficulty breathing with indigestion, belching, burping and hiccupping. They might also pass a lot of wind but with no relief. The ethereal soul is responsible for our state of mind a. subconscious when we sleep and therefore determines our dreams. With a full stomach, you may have vivid dreams, sleepwalking, sleep talking, and dreaming the same dream, and most of the time these dreams are not nice. Sometimes when you wake up you are physically crying. This is related to a total detachment between the physical body and the soul, spirit, mind, and subconscious. People will often describe their experience as being out of the body.

2. Stores the Blood

The Liver stores the blood according to the physical activity of the human, and from a female aspect according to the time of the month concerning the period or ovulation.

The Progesterone is yang. Yang has the aspect of pushing, moving, and warming. The Progesterone and yang are responsible for starting the period at the right time because of their pushing and movement function. When the progesterone rises this means yang is rising and can lead to headaches or irritability. Oestrogen is yin. The function of Oestrogen and yin is to cool and moisture, to prepare the reproductive system for fertility.

When you move you need oxygen. This physical activity needs the work of three organs at the same time, the Lungs take oxygen, the Heart circulates the oxygen to the working muscles, and the Liver produces the glucose the glycogen to the working muscles. The Liver is responsible for starting the Period. This means any woman who has a late period, heavy period, irregular, scanty period, no period, or getting more than one period a month, from an oriental perspective their Liver will have a part to play in it. Women should not have any period symptoms at all. If the Liver ensures the smooth flow of qi and the Liver releases the period from the storage at the right time of the month then the woman will not have the following symptoms: Back Pain, Headaches, Bloatedness, Nausea, Irritability Mood Swings, and Tender Breast (especially the left breast).

From an oriental perspective, the Liver is yin and the Gallbladder is yang. The Liver channel ends on the side of the ribs below the breast. From an oriental perspective, the Heart captures the mind. This explains why some women have breast milk and they cannot express it. A mammogram will show nothing at all, or the result will be inconclusive. The explanation for this from an oriental perspective is because the Liver holds the aspect of anger, hatred, resentment, frustration. The more women hold these emotions the more stagnant her qi and her blood will become especially on the left breast. The Heart carries the emotional aspect and the Liver is responsible for the spark and starting the emotional aspect. Women who breastfeed their children for at least two years for five to ten minutes a day are, from an oriental perspective, not only physically supplying the milk and nutrients to the baby but it is also an emotional process that gives love, affection, and tenderness all at the same time. It is a purification process. The woman is purifying her body and she is giving the baby a natural antibiotic and at the same time, she is releasing any emotional aspect through the process.

Some people ask if this means the mother is passing her emotions to the baby. The answer is no. However, by opening the milk duct and the channel will help the aspect of letting go. If you take children as an example, when they fight with each other they will be playing with each other once again after five or ten minutes, because generally speaking the adults are the ones who hold grudges and keep their anger and hatred regardless of what the reason for it is.

Heavy Periods

Generally speaking, a heavy period is related to yang deficiency. The function of the yang is to push upward and warm. The blood is regarded as an organ and has to stay in the vessels. If there is a yang deficiency this means the blood is not able to be 'held in the place where it should be'. This could be due to any of the following:

- Heart yang deficiency
- Kidney yang deficiency
- Spleen yang deficiency

Heart yang deficiency means the, is cold in the body especially with bad circulation. It might exist with excess yin. This also explains why anything we eat or drink that is below is below room temperature will affect the Heart and will also affect the Kidney and the Spleen but especially the Spleen as it will undermine the Spleen function because the Spleen is the only organ in the human body that has to push the energy upward from toes to the head. Heavy periods can also be related to Kidney yang deficiency. This is because the Kidney's open into the three orifices and of course the period has to pass through the vagina. If there is yang deficiency this is one of the reasons the period will be very heavy.

Scanty Periods

This is related to the function of the Liver by ensuring the smooth flow of Qi to start the period at the right time. It is also related and linked to other aspects, for example, if this woman has anaemia and does not eat a well-balanced diet and does not have enough nutrients this will mean that the body is lacking in Iron, in the first place and the body will not be able to push and start the period. If the period does start it will be very short and very scanty. A woman could be anaemic and also have heavy periods, bruise easily, and have a poor healing mechanism. This might be related to other reasons such as fibroids, adhesion, endometriosis, or cysts. From an oriental perspective, it could also be due to any form of sexual disease and this will make matters worse.

Irregular Periods

Generally speaking, this is related to a hormonal imbalance. From an oriental perspective, it is related to your emotional state and the state of your mind.

Painful Periods

This is caused by a stagnation of Liver qi, especially in the reproductive system. When Liver Qi is stagnant every part of your body will pay the price. This explains why women get headaches with their period. The reason for this is because the Liver qi is stagnant and cannot supply enough oxygen, blood, and glucose to the brain. Women may also have back pain and tender breasts. The back is covered by a large number of muscles. Generally speaking, muscles need a huge supply of energy, oxygen, and fluid such as potassium, calcium, magnesium, and sodium so that they can function to their optimum level of health and wellbeing. If Liver Qi is stagnant the muscles on the back will not receive all of what was mentioned above, and this will lead to spasm, stiffness, cramps, and general backache particularly the lower back. The same principle can be applied to pin down the legs. The muscles on the front of the body also need the same amount of oxygen, blood, and fluids mentioned above, and the woman will have bloatedness, nausea, cramps, diarrhea, and spasms. These come like waves. Sometimes the woman will also pass a lot of wind. In some cases, the muscles are so tensed and cramped up and stiff. In this case, if the pain is related to excess and you put your hand on the area and you press it, it makes the condition ten times worse. For example, if you have a migraine or vertigo and your head is pounding and your heart is beating very fast and you press your head you will make it worse because you are adding excess to excess. If the pain is related to deficiency regardless of whether it is yin or yang and you put your hand on the painful area you will feel a sense of relief and comfort, but it does not solve the problem. From an oriental perspective, the human touch has healing power and a reassuring aspect to it. Sometimes people will go to the doctor because of the pain and discomfort and the doctor will prescribe painkillers or anti-inflammatory medication. This medication will sometimes relieve all the physical symptoms such as cramps, spasms, headaches, etc. However, from an oriental perspective, the person will still have the emotional and psychological aspect which is embedded down to the person's cellular and tissue level. This is what we mean when we say, 'your issue is in your tissue'. The state of your mind will add and will reflect on the severity of your physical condition regardless of what it is and whether the person is male or female. For example, sometimes when people have pain, they start to become anxious and worry about the pain.

They might worry they have cancer. When the doctor tells the person that everything is fine, and they have nothing to worry about this reassures the person and the person's mind will be at peace and this will start the healing process and recovery state.

The Liver will release the blood according to the time of the month. If Live qi is flowing smoothly and freely the period will start at the right time and ovulation will take place at the right time and vice versa. The first thing we need to do for women who are struggling with infertility is to regulate their period so that they know their time of ovulation. This will increase their likelihood of becoming pregnant.

A woman's painful period could be caused by anger and another's caused by fear and another's by shock and the list is endless. This explains why their treatment and the combination of acupuncture needles used will be different as also will the emotional and physical exercise given to them. As we mentioned earlier, if six people go to the doctor with a headache they will receive the same tablet because from a western perspective the medication is designed for us before we have the condition, for example, inhaler for asthma, cream for eczema, laxatives for constipation and the list is endless. The prescribed medication will deal with the manifestation however the ailment may come back again. From an oriental perspective, the example above using the six women and their period can be applied to any medical condition, the title of the complaint is the same however the treatment is different because we go to the root cause of the condition and we don't just deal with the manifestation.

As we said, from an oriental perspective the tongue and the pulse will determine a person's emotional state and will get deep down to the emotional root cause of the problem which will, in turn, contribute to a person's physical complaint. From an oriental perspective, emotions are compared to the layers of an onion. For example, if one person has chronic arthritis for thirty years and another person has acute arthritis from a twisted ankle, one is a chronic emotional problem caused by sadness and grief and the other is an acute emotion from sadness and grief. Of course, it will take longer to treat the person who has thirty years of sadness. It will also depend on what chakra is affected and on what channel and what organ is paying the price and it is also related to the environment the person lives in and the people they live with. If a person is depressed and sad and three other people in the family are depressed, then the situation will be made worse because you are feeding each other's emotions and negativity.

3. Manifests in the Nails

Healthy nails should be shiny and glowing. There should be no sign of blue, black, or brown colours on the nail. They should not be too thin and they should not break easily and they should grow at a normal rate. If you have dark or black nails it is due to stagnation of Liver qi, regardless of what the reason for the stagnation is, whether it is emotional due to holding anger, hatred, frustration, resentment or whether it is stagnation due to a lack of blood and iron and you are anaemic from the first place. Another form of stagnation is related to the overconsumption of icy cold drinks which will affect the circulation and therefore your nails will not receive the necessary blood and nutrients to nourish them. Anything below room temperature will affect our heart from a western perspective and the circulation also, and it will undermine the Spleen from an oriental perspective. As we said earlier, the Spleen is the only organ in the body, from an oriental perspective, that has to push the energy against gravity from the sole of the feet to the top of the head twenty-four hours a day. This means the Spleen from an oriental perspective represents the Heart and circulation from a western perspective. This means the venous return of blood. If your nails are thin, dry, and cracked and they break easily it is a sign of a lack of vitamins, minerals, and nutrients in general and over a long period, this will affect the hair on your head.

There are a variety of reasons for weakness in the nails:

> It could be due to an injury to the nails. Generally speaking, this is not a good indication. You will rarely injure all your nails. One example would be due to the use of chemical substances

> Using medication over a long period will destroy, ruin or damage them which in turn will make your nails dry.

> In some cases, people who are undergoing treatment for cancer will find that the treatment affects the hair on their body and their nails also. This will depend on what type of chemotherapy treatment you are having and the aggression of cancer.

> People who swim regularly, over a long period, might find the chemical in the water affect their nails.

From an oriental perspective, when all of these physical injuries are excluded, you must look at the emotional state of the person and how they feel and think as this will reflect upon their circulation. The Liver ensures the smooth flow of qi and stores the blood. If qi is stagnant due to emotional reasons this will affect the quality of the nails and it will also affect your sight as a sense. When qi is stagnant blood will also be stagnant and when the blood is stagnant it is unable to reach your extremities, the furthest of which are the nails on the fingers and toes

Your general diet and fluid intake can also affect the weaknesses and abnormalities of the nail. A diet that does not contain enough vitamins and minerals will affect the quality of the nails. Most people who have anaemia and are lacking in iron will have brittle and weak nails. A diet lacking in Calcium, Potassium, Magnesium, or Sodium will also cause weak and abnormal nails as these substances and nutrients represent the yin and the yang: Calcium is yang – Magnesium is yin, Sodium is yang – Potassium is yin

If the nail condition and weakness are related to diet then the person should be covering the five elements from a nutrient and oriental perspective. These are: Carbohydrate, Protein, Fat, Minerals, and Vitamins, Fluids

The vitamins, minerals, and fluids are especially important daily. For example, six pieces of fruit, taken two at a time three times daily but not on an empty stomach, will help to lead a balanced diet. This matches the saying 'an apple a day keeps the doctor away'. This is because the apple can neutralize the acid to make it alkaline. Generally speaking, ninety-nine per cent of our health problems are related to our stomach as an organ which is responsible for the digestion as a process and to our excretion as bowel and the kidney and urinary bladder as urine. The stomach and the bowel represent the immune system from an oriental perspective and a western perspective also and will determine your health and well-being in general. Very good digestion and excretion system is the secret to a very healthy person in general. The secret to a healthy digestion and excretion system is drinking plenty o water especially first thing in the morning when you wake up, ideally two to three glasses. filtered water is a form of water that does not contain fluoride and chloride and is a good alternative to tap water. Drinking water twenty minutes before every meal will also help digestion. The more acid we have in the body the more trouble we will have. The Stomach is a source of acid in the form of gastric juices. If there is too much acid, there will be dryness as the acid will dry the fluids.

To look at it from a different perspective, seventy per cent of our body is made up of fluids, two-thirds of the world is fluid. The cell cannot function without the fluid. The cell has to go through five functions down to a cellular level to make our health reach its optimum level of health and wellbeing. These five functions are part of the theory of five elements and as I always keep mentioning the world is built on the yin and yang and the five elements from every perspective.

The cells have to do the following functions:

1) The cell is permeable. It has to allow the transportation and transformation of fluid between cell to cell and tissue to tissue, up to organ level and system and human level.
2) The cell has to extract the energy from the food you eat. This is called ATP Adenosine Triphosphate.
3) The cell has to take oxygen.
4) The cell has to expel carbon dioxide and any form of waste product such as uric and lactic acid.
5) The cell has to die when their time is up and they have to be replaced by a new cell which has to do the same function for a certain period which is determined by what type of cell it is and what function it has to do and what tissue and organ it belongs to because every cell has a different life span.

The function of your body down to the cellular level determines your health and wellbeing in general and especially the quality of your nails.

4. Controls the Sinews

The word sinews means ligament, cartilage, and tendon.

The ligament is a tough band of tissue. It connects bone to bone. The best example of a ligament is the cruciate ligament in the knee. The cruciate ligament is inside your knees and connects the thigh bone (Femur) to the lower limb (Tibia and Fibula).

The tendon is made up of tough bands of tissue that come together to form the tendon. It connects muscle to bone. An example of a tendon is the Achilles tendon which connects the calf muscle located on the back of the lower leg (called Gastrocnemius) and the muscle below the calf muscle but above the heel (called Soleus) to the bone at the back of the heel (called Calcaneus).

The cartilage is also made up of tough bands of tissue. Cartilage lies between the joints and acts as a cushion, similar to a sponge, and prevents friction between bones and aids with the free and smooth movement of the joint. The best way to describe it by comparing it to the clutch in a car, you cannot drive the car with your foot constantly on the clutch. The clutch has the same function as the cartilage, to provide the cushion to prevent friction between metal and metal.

The sinews connect all our joints to our muscles. When you move, whether you walk, jog, swim, or perform any physical activity you need the ligament, tendon, and cartilage. They all work together as one unit so that you can do the movement. The older we get the less elasticity we will have, and the ligament, cartilage, and tendons will decrease and shrink in their shape and size. This explains why the movements we were able to do when we were twenty are not as easy for us to do when we are fifty as we do have the same range of motion. Apart from the aging process affecting the sinews, there are a variety of other reasons for them to be affected:

> ## *Using the joint incorrectly*

Using the joint incorrectly will speed up the process of degeneration. Standing, sitting, walking, or moving incorrectly will harm the sinews. It is not unusual to see someone aged twenty-five and they have knee problems or need a knee replacement. People who walk with their toes pointing out generally speaking will have trouble with their knees and may have a knee replacement. People who walk with their toes pointing, generally speaking, will have problems with their hips and may need a hip replacement. This is because the joint is out of the midline and out of alignment. Before doing any physical activity, the posture should be mastered. When doing physical activity such as walking or jogging, imagine that you have three shoes, the third shoe being in the middle between the left and right shoes. This third shoe is imaginary and you use this image to keep you straight and aligned. The small toe should be in a straight line with the ankle. The knee has to land in front of you when you walk without the toes turning out or in. When you stand and bend the knees like you are sitting in a pretend chair position the knees should land immediately on your toes. This is a medical sign from anatomy and psychological perspective that the joints are in the right direction. For example, you cannot drive the car with the tyres pointing out. The same applies to the joints. A good indication is to look at your old shoes and see what part of the shoe is worn. If the shoe is worn from the side from the small toe to the heel this means that you are more likely to suffer from hip problems as the toes are pointing in when you move. If the shoe is worn from the side from the big toe to the arch and the inside heel this means you are more likely to suffer from knee problems as the toes are pointing out when you move. The same process which is taking place in the shows, being the grinding and wearing, is also taking place in the sinews and all that will be left is bone against bone.

➢ *Consuming a lot of sugary foods and alcohol*

When the ligaments, tendons, cartilage, and tissues do not receive enough lubricant it will lead to tightness and dryness of the joint and all the connected tissue. The lubricant is not being provided because carbohydrates and sugar create heat which dries up the fluids.

➢ *Drugs and Chemicals*

Using drugs and chemicals over a long period will destroy and demolish the yin. The yin has the function to cool and moisture and to provide lubricant which is equivalent to the body fluid in general but in this case the synovial fluid. The best way to describe the synovial fluid is by comparing it to the white of an egg. The fluid has to be slimy to provide the lubricant and the moisture aspect to the joint. If a person is continuously and repetitively carrying out the same movement the fluid will turn from being slimy to runny. Over a long period, the fluid will become inflamed resulting in a condition called synovitis. In some cases, the inflammation can be so severe that it needs to be drained. The repetitive movement is not giving the fluid the chance to renew and to replenish itself and to make enough moisture and lubricant for the next day.

➢ *Diet*

Not eating a well-balanced diet can affect your sinews. A well-balanced diet should contain the five elements which form a nutritional perspective are: Carbohydrate, Protein, Fats, Vitamins, and Minerals, Fluid.

Anaemia is a condition where the body is lacking in iron. This will affect the joints and sinews and will also affect the eyes because as we now know, the Liver opens into the eyes. Too much iron is called Hemochromatosis and leads to loss of flexibility. Having too much iron can be compared to compacted cement which has no space for movement and expansion. This leads to tightness and stiffness along with cramps and spasms of the joint and muscle. This will also lead to too much pressure on the head and eyes and clients often describe it as feeling like their head and eyeballs are going to explode. The person will look very tense and very red. Too much iron in the body will lead to dryness especially in the stomach and in the bowel and will lead to constipation. Sometimes the excess iron arises from excessive consumption of iron however in some cases the person could be vegetarian and yet the iron level is still high. In this case, it is caused by the Liver and because it is produced by the Liver it will interfere with the smooth flow of Qi and because the Qi does not flow freely the person will have stiffness, spasms, and tightness. Physical movement will be difficult and it will also be difficult to get into a comfortable position in bed with twisting and turning.

5. Opens into the Eyes

As I mentioned earlier the Liver is a yin organ and its paired organ, the Gallbladder, is a yang organ. From an oriental perspective, every five-element organ is related to a sense and in the case of the Liver, the eyes are the related sense. The sense of sigh is the mediator between the inside and the outside world. From an oriental perspective the eye and the sense of sight is related to the physical makeup and anatomy and physiology of the eyes such as the iris and the pupil, instead, it is related to your internal thoughts and to the state of your mind, especially the spiritual state and the state which is related to your soul and spirit. This coincides with the saying 'the eyes are the window of the soul'. As we said, the soul is the picture and the spirit is the frame. This means the spirit has to contain the soul. If the soul and the spirit are not grounded and the person's mind is wandering from subject to subject and from idea to idea, the person will have excessive and rapid eye movement and excessive and rapid blinking, as if the person is unable to control their eyes.

The Liver energy flows similar to that of waves. The waves of energy come in a sudden, abrupt, and impulsive manner and can lead to twitching in the eyes and jerking and jumping of eye muscles. There are of course other reasons from an anatomy and physiology perspective that would cause the same problems. Our eyes should be surrounded by fluid, which is the tear. The taste of the tear is salty. The eyelid is a form of protection and preserves the eyes. Moist eyes are always better than dry eyes. The tears are fluid, they represent the yin aspect, and the function of the tear is the function of the yin, to cool and moisture. If there is too much heat in the eyes it will dry up the fluid and will result in itchy, irritated, dry, and red eyes. Sometimes with age, this might lead to cataracts or detached retina. The link between the Liver and the eyes is as follows:

The Liver releases blood and glycogen to all our organs and also to all our senses including the eyes. If a person consumes a lot of carbohydrates and sweet food the eyes and the sight will be the first organ and sense to pay the price. The eyes have very tiny hair-like threads called capillaries whose job it is to carry the oxygen, fluid, nutrients, and glucose to the eyes. Too much sugar and fat will lead to a blockage in these capillaries resulting in the flow of oxygen, fluid, nutrients, and glucose being obstructed. When the Liver function, as a yin organ, is impaired then its paired yang organ, the Gallbladder, the function will also be impaired and will be unable to break down the fats. This will result in an accumulation of sugar in the blood and an accumulation of a fatty substance called cholesterol in the veins, arteries, and capillaries. This in turn will affect all of our body and senses including the eyes.

The medical name for having too much cholesterol is Arterial Sclerosis and means hardening of the artery wall. This is not always related to your diet. Sometimes a person's diet could be perfect or they could be vegetarian but yet they still high cholesterol and a high sugar level. This because the Liver is producing more fat than the body needs. The Liver can also produce more iron than the body needs resulting in a condition called Hemochromatosis. These will accumulate and will invade the body and especially the sight. The more iron and fat that you have the more your sight will pay the price. Symptoms include a feeling of pressure in the head and eyes, often described as a feeling of being ready to explode. The iron will also dry up all the body fluid including the fluid in the eyes and the bowel resulting in dry, brown, and hard stools. Over a long period, this will lead to a dark stool and sometimes occasional bleeding during defecation. If the blood is bright red during the bowel motion this might be bleeding through the external tissue and could be related to Haemorrhoids and might not be too serious. However, if the blood is dark brown and mixed with the bowel motion, this is more likely coming from tissue deep inside and can be a sign of a more serious issue. Should this turn to cancer is will result in a process of consumption, the yin consuming the yang and the yang consuming the yin, and can be seen in alterations between bowel movements, having diarrhea, and then constipation. There may be a frequent need to move the bowels however after the motion it may feel like you need to move the bowels and you di not empty enough. The bowel should be a moist environment for defecation. The stool should move easily and smoothly.

The link between the Liver, the bowel, and the eyes is that all three of them hold the aspect of letting go and detoxifying the body:

- ➤ The function of the Liver is to detoxify the body – letting go.
- ➤ The function of the bowel is defecation which is expelling toxins from inside the body to the outside – this is the structural aspect of letting go. Constipation over a long period can lead to cancer.
- ➤ You cry through the eyes. Crying is a process of purification and detoxification from the emotional aspect especially anger, hatred, resentment, frustration and jealously.

As I mentioned earlier there are three types of crying. You cry when you are sad, and this is related to your Lungs as an organ. Sometimes you cry when you are happy, and this is related to the Heart as an organ. The third type is you cry whether you are happy or sad and this is related to your Liver as an organ. If Liver Qi is stagnated and does not flow freely you will reach a stage where you will not be able to cry at all no matter how much you try and you might feel a 'lump like sensation in your throat, similar to an emotional tumor, and also a heavy burden in the chest. From an oriental perspective, there are special points to open the water passages and which will make the client cry. Some clients will cry immediately, and some will cry when they go home. When the water passages are open it holds the aspect of letting go. This is a different form of crying and is not related to being happy or sad. The points used are LU7, S.16, SP9, and REN9. At the time of the treatment, depending on whether the client is feeling warm or cold, you use REN6 to heat the body or REN4 to cool the body. If the client is cold, they have yang deficiency, the function of yang is to warm and push, and they will have no power to push to cry. They will be unable to push the tears out due to the yang deficiency and they will feel like an obstacle or barrier is preventing them from crying. In this case, they have enough tears but no power to push the tears; this is ninety-nine percent emotional. If the client is hot the heat will dry up the clients' tears. As mentioned earlier the eyes need to be immersed in a fluid and when the fluid is gone dryness will ensue. In this case, you need to know how the fluid dried up because it did not happen overnight. If a person drinks a lot of alcohol especially vodka and whiskey, the Liver has to work very hard to detoxify the body. In this case, the eyes will be deprived of the nutrients and fluids which they are supposed to receive continuously and which are provided to the eyes via the movement of Liver qi from an oriental perspective and with the help of the heart's circulation the Lungs respiration actions from a western perspective. If you look at the eyes of a drunk person, they will look red, dry, bloodshot, and sometimes protruded. To look at it in another way, alcohol contains a lot of sugar. The sugar will abuse the eyes and it will destroy the sight. People with Diabetes will often have bad eyesight. You will often hear of people who cannot drink a lot of alcohol without first consuming heavy food which contains a lot of carbohydrates, to 'soak up' the alcohol. This is a recipe for disaster and can be described as added fuel to the fire. The treatment is about plenty of fluid, avoiding sugar and alcohol, nourishing the fluids, and bringing the fluid up to the eyes through pulling the yang up (DU20). The tip of the nose could also be needled or tapped, this will open the tear duct and the sinus and will bring tears to the eyes and as I mentioned earlier the sinus is the first gate to the respiratory system. If, when you wake in the morning, you don't have 'sleep' in your eyes this means that the eyes have not been regenerated overnight and a new cell has not been created. If you don't sleep, you may have a lesser life expectancy because certain cells need to regenerate. Daytime is yang. When your eyes are open in the daytime, they are in a yang state because the blinking and movement action is yang. Yang is hollow and has space and when the eyes are open, they need space. Night-time is yin, yin is dense and compact. The fluid in the eyes is yin. When your eyes are closed they are dense and compact. This explains why if you do not sleep due to working night shifts or if you suffer from insomnia for a long period you will have itchy, irritated, and dry eyes along with back circles under the eyes. This is because during the sleeping process the fluid will be purified and regenerated to prepare the eyes for the next day. The 'sleep' in your eyes when you wake up along with a salty taste in your mouth is a residue of the cells and fluid regenerating and means that the eyes have produced enough lubricant for their function the next day and the stomach has also produced enough gastric juices as a lubricant for the digestion process the next day. The link between the stomach and the eyes is the stomach channel starts at Stomach 1 immediately under the eyelids. The Stomachs paired yin organ, the Spleen, controls the sweet taste. In years gone by a traditional check-up to determine if you were anaemic or lacking in nutrients was to pull down the lower eyelid to check the colour. This check gives a general indication about your health in general and especially your eyes and stomach.

6. Controls the Ethereal Soul

From an oriental perspective, the Liver controls the ethereal soul. As I mentioned earlier, the Lungs control the corporeal soul which is responsible for our actions behaviours when we are awake. The corporeal soul controls the way we walk, talk, stand, think, behave, and feel while we are awake. It is related to our sympathetic nervous system from a western perspective. The sympathetic nervous system is related to our physical body and its physical movement, balance, and coordination. The corporeal soul represents our state of alertness and being awake which is opposite to our state of being asleep and unconscious which is controlled by the liver. The ethereal soul is responsible for our actions and behavior while we are sleeping and while we are attached deep down to the cellular level and our subconscious, heart, and spirit. The word ether means air. The ethereal soul travels through the night, like travelling in the air. It goes wandering and does not have any plan or any sense of direction. It is spaceless, weightless, and timeless. The best way to describe it is like someone going to the airport and they don't know the name or time of their flight or the country they are travelling to. They don't know where they are going but yet they want to travel. The Gallbladder is the paired yang organ with the Liver. The Gallbladder is responsible for our sense of judgment without hesitation and it gives us the sense of direction whether it be physical direction related to our right, light, up and down or directions to the place we want to travel to, or the sense of direction related to our decision making. The Gallbladder helps us to make the right decision at the right time at the right moment. For example, you go to buy a new house and the estate agents show you ten houses. This is the time when the Gallbladder helps you to choose the best house you would like to live in and make your home and means you have no sense of hesitation or confusion so that later you will not regret the decision you have made. It is interesting to note that clients who have had their Gallbladder removed will often comment that their judgment is not the same as it was before the Gallbladder being removed, that it takes them a longer period to think and reflect on a simple decision. This is concerning anything and not only about houses. The Gallbladder is responsible for this state of decision making not only when we awake but also when we are asleep. If you plan for the next day, for example, that you will wake up at 7 am, have breakfast at 7.20 am, leave for work at 8 am, etc. Verbally these decisions have been made but as an action, they are still in a transitional state. These actions are still a part of your subconscious state and are embedded down to the cellular level. The next day the Liver will ensure the smooth flow of qi and the Gallbladder will give you a sense of direction and the kidneys will give you the motivation to act upon what you have planned. If the Gallbladder function is in harmony with the Liver, you will have pleasant dreams because the Gallbladder will give the ethereal soul the sense of direction and clarity which is needed deep down to the cellular level. If the Gallbladder does not work in harmony with the Liver and does not provide a sense of direction to the ethereal soul, then the ethereal soul will go wandering and you will have vivid dreams, unpleasant dreams, and repetitive dreams, There may also be sleepwalking, sleep talking or an inability to find a comfortable position in bed. You might find that you wake up every morning at the same time and either you can't go back to sleep at all or it takes a long time to fall back asleep.

There are twenty-four hours in the day and there are twelve channels in the body, six yin, and six yang. Every two hours the energy passes from a yin channel to the yang channel. The time at which the dream takes place will determine the disconnection and the detachment between the liver and the gallbladder as a yin and yang channel and also the affected and connected channel. For example, the Lungs are related to sadness and grief, if the dream takes place at the same time the energy is passing through the Lung channel the dream will be sad and you might cry in the dream or wake up with tears in your eyes. Our dreams are also related to the Heart which captures the Mind and takes us to the subconscious stage to give us a peaceful night's sleep. From an oriental perspective, the Blood is considered to be an organ and is responsible for capturing the Mind. Eating too much sugar or iron before bed will affect the quality of your sleep and will also affect your dreams.

If you know how to train your mind and create the link between the soul, the spirit, the mind, and the subconscious, and if you have access to your subconscious you will be able to dream the type of dream you want to dream. When you learn how to link with the subconscious the process will become easier. Generally speaking, this process will not happen overnight as it needs a lot of training and practice. Concentration and meditation is the first step to start this process and the process also needs complete silence and quiet. You can also re-wire the circuit in your brain by using repetition over and over. For example, if you wake up at 4 am every morning to pray or meditate this will become a habit, and eventually, you will wake up at 4 am even if you don't need to wake. From a western perspective, this is called the brain clock. By linking the brain clock with the action you want to do you will then be able to dream the dream you want to dream.

CHAPTER 4

PATTERNS OF THE LIVER

Stagnation of Liver Qi

This condition is caused by the stagnation of the liver over a long period which subsequently leads to mental and emotional strain. Liver qi can become stagnant in all of the body in general but especially in the liver channel due to hatred, anger, resentment, frustration and jealousy. These are the emotions that prevent the liver qi from flowing freely and smoothly. When liver qi is stagnated, it will stop moving and because the liver qi is responsible for moving the qi of all the organs this means that the other organs and channels will pay the price for the liver qi stagnation.

Liver qi can also become stagnant due to physical reasons such as injury or consuming a lot of alcohol or drugs. Smoking will also affect the smooth flow of qi. When liver qi is stagnated, it will affect each organ and area that the liver channel passed through.

Signs and symptoms:

1)   Hypochondriac pain.

The liver channel passes through the hypochondriac region and the digestive area and when qi is stagnated in this are it can result in pain and discomfort.

2)   Heaviness and discomfort in the chest due to the liver channel passing through the area

3) Breast pain and discomfort in females which becomes worse during the pre-menstrual stage, ovulation and menstruation.

Generally speaking, both breasts will be affected by the stagnation of Liver qi however the left breast will be more affected due to the location above the heart and the pericardium, the muscular sac surrounding the heart, which holds all our emotions. When women experience tender breasts during and/or before their period this is due to the fluctuation of their hormones from an anatomy and physiology perspective and the stagnation of liver qi from ana oriental perspective.

4) Emotional fluctuations before, and/or during menstruation

The stagnation of the liver qi will determine how the woman feels, acts and reacts before and/or during menstruation. It is often the case that around the time of menstruation a woman might laugh at something one minute and cry at it the next. This is because the liver qi is like the waves of the ocean and can be compared to an emotional electrocardiogram.

When the liver qi is moving away from the body you will laugh but when the liver qi is invading the body it will add to the hormonal imbalance and also to the state of instability which makes the matter worse.

5) Bloating, belching, hiccup and heartburn

This is because the liver channel passes through the digestive area and when it is stagnated in this area it will interfere with the direct flow of qi in the digestive area especially the stomach. Stomach qi descends, when you eat the food has to go down, when liver qi is stagnated here it will not allow the food to descend down and instead, the food will come back up and will bring acid with it. The same can be applied to the lung Qi if liver qi invades lung qi the lung qi will not be able to descend when you breathe in and it will be either stagnant in the chest causing headaches and difficulty breathing and sighing or it will cause a build-up or air resulting in hiccups and belching. From an oriental perspective, this caused rebellious stomach qi and rebellious lung qi.

6)   Accumulation of phlegm and damp especially in the throat. Stagnation of liver Qi over a long period along with rebellious stomach qi leads to the accumulation of phlegm and damp, especially in the throat. It is often described as having a lump or stone in the throat and can make the person unable to speak or they will speak in a weak, shallow and weepy voice and may affect the swallowing of food. From an oriental perspective, this is regarded as an emotional tumour of the throat and oesophagus. Over a long period, this emotional tumour may turn into a physical tumour and the physical tumour will produce the same symptoms as the emotional tumour produced which are:

a) Difficulty breathing
b) Difficulty swallowing food
c) Difficulty drinking
d) Hoarseness of the voice
e) Rapid pulse and rapid loss of appetite
f) Rapid loss of body weight

Liver Fire Blazing Upwards

This condition is caused by stagnation of liver qi for a long period. The main emotions which cause liver qi to stagnate are hatred, anger, resentment, frustration and jealously. It can also be caused by psychological strain and by drinking alcohol and smoking which will demolish the yin in general but especially liver yin. The function of yin is to cool and provide moisture, in this condition these aspects no longer exist which results in heat building up in the body. This heat over a long period will turn into fire. This fire will rise and blaze upwards, especially in the liver channel. Fire is yang in nature and yang will rise towards the face and the head.

Signs and symptoms:

➢ Dizziness and distending sensation in the head, headache

This can feel like the head is ready to explode because the liver fire which goes up towards the head causes hyperactivity in the head hence the dizziness, distension and headache.

➢ Dry, itchy, irritated eyes

From an oriental perspective, the liver opens into the eyes. Liver fire will dry up liver yin which means that there is no cooling moistening aspect, especially in the eyes. From an oriental perspective, the liver yin represents the tear of the eyes and the tear duct from a western perspective. If there are not enough tears produced, due to dryness caused by the liver fire blazing towards the head and face but especially the eyes or due to a structural blockage in the tear duct which may have been caused by an injury such as a broken nose or skull or by an overgrowth of pollen inside the nose or inside the tear duct which prevents the tear from being produced in the first place or prevents the tear from flowing smoothly, this will result in dry, red and itchy eyes. Sometimes only one side is blocked and when the person cries, they feel the tears are not produced equally and evenly. Subsequently, this will affect eyesight in general.

People who wear glasses will find that the stronger the glasses are the more they will squint and frown. When you squint you are blocking your third eye chakra which is located between the eyebrows. This will affect your focus, concentration, memory and perception. When your third eye is blocked it will also affect your lungs and breathing in general. The capacity of the lungs to take in the air will be reduced. Also, the squinting and frowning will result in a lack of blood supply to the brain. The eyes have capillaries which carry oxygen, fluid and nutrients around the eyes, squinting and frowning will also affect the function of these capillaries resulting in a lack of fluids and oxygen reaching the eyes.

➢ Red and dry face. Sometimes only the cheeks will be red.

➢ Bloodshot eyes or in severe cases, bleeding from the eyes.

The liver can be so intense that it rises into the head and the eyes. If the person's ankles are twisted this will affect the sight as a sense and the eyes and also the hearing as a sense and the ears and sometimes may lead to migraine and vertigo. A twisted ankle causes the vision and the hearing on the same side to pay the price.

➢ Bleeding from the eyes or nose or both

This is caused by intense liver fire and wind which puts a huge amount of pressure on the anterior wall of the arteries and capillaries. When these arteries and capillaries are not able to cope with this pressure they start to rupture. The capillaries are so small in size and shape that they are not able to cope with this pressure. The consequences of this will be either bleeding from the eyes, nose or both. This can be a common occurrence in children who have a habit of picking their nose or it can also happen when there is a direct blow to the nose or eyes but especially the nose, or when the weather is hot and humid and the intensity of the heat will cause the bleeding particularly from the nose.

➢ Bitter taste or bitter and sour taste in the mouth and throat. This is caused by hyperactivity of the liver fire and liver wind at the same time.

➢ Feeling angry or frustrated. The person becomes angry, frustrated and upset very easily.

This is because anger is the emotion linked and connected to the liver as an organ and the liver as a channel. Each structure that the liver channel passes through from start to finish will be affected and will pay the price for this anger. Generally speaking, anger, resentment, frustration, hatred and jealousy which are generated by liver fire and liver wind will lead to stiffness, cramps, spasms and sinews which become tight and rigid and will shrink in size and shape which in turn will affect the flexibility of the joint and muscles and movement will be difficult. Every movement will become difficult to do regardless of whether the person is lying in bed and they will find it difficult to find a comfortable position to lie in and will keep twisting and turning. To encourage a peaceful nights sleep it is recommended to do the following:

a) Don't go to bed with a full stomach
b) It is important to"wind-down" before going to bed either by meditating, praying or hypnosis

c) Deep and slow breathing is essential for the process to take place
d) Drink a lot of water throughout the day especially first thing in the morning to wash the body's systems and organs from the acidity and toxins that go through it during the day. The more neutralised and alkaline the body is and toxin-free, the better the body will function and the easier the sleeping will be
e) Contemplation and visualisation that you are in the sleeping stage even before going to bed helps also
f) Chanting a spiritual prayer, especially silently, with yourself allows you to access your subconscious which is very important for the sleeping process to take place from start to finish
g) Avoid watching violent films before bed as these will create hyperactivity
h) If you find it difficult to visualise, contemplate or hypnotise yourself your practitioner will be able to give you a programme designed for you as an individual to practice at home to help you to have a peaceful nights sleep.
i) The tongue coating will be yellow because the heat has accumulated and turns into damp heat.
j) The pulse will be very wiry and rapid because heat and wind together cause hyperactivity hence the fast and rapid pulse.

Stagnation of Cold in the Liver Channel

This condition is caused by the invasion of the liver as an organ and the liver as a channel by either external or internal cold. External cold can derive from drinking cold drinks or eating food which is below room temperature or from exposure to damp, cold or wet weather. This cold from the external environment will settle in the internal environment. The cold will invade the body in general but especially the spleen, kidney and liver channels. An example of people who will be affected by the invasion of cold is the farmers who work in the wet, cold and damp rice fields. The cold will invade the channel through the external environment and will pass through the channel and will affect each structure, area and organ which the channel passes through. As the liver channel circles the reproductive system and passes through the abdomen area in both the male and female body these areas will be affected directly and immediately by the invasion of the cold in the liver channel.

Signs and symptoms:

➤ Lower abdominal pain, bloating and distended stomach.
➤ This is because the cold invasion causes contraction, cramping and spasm in the abdomen, excretion and reproductive areas. The contraction and spasm are caused by stagnation of qi and blood in these areas.
➤ Swelling and distension of the testicles and scrotum.
➤ The person will have a dragging and damp sensation of the testicle and scrotum from a male aspect.
➤ Women will have a white vaginal discharge along with a bearing down pain in the lower abdomen area. This can sometimes be worse during ovulation or before and during menstruation.

The reason for this is because when the cold invades the liver channel the liver will be no longer able to smooth the free flow of qi. As a result, qi will become stagnant and because qi pushes blood to warm the body and blood nourishes qi for the energy, when qi is stagnated by the invasion of cold in the liver channel this leads to further cold which will become residual in all of the channels and affected structures and organs. Qi is yang in nature and blood is yin in nature and because the function of the yang is to push and warm-up the circulation in all of our body hence the person will have a yang deficiency which is caused by the invasion of the liver channel by cold.

In this case, the person might also have spleen yang deficiency and kidney yang deficiency. The Ren channel passes through the front of the body and is yin in nature and represents the cold aspect. The opposite channel to the Ren is the Du channel which is on the back of the body on the spine and represents the yang aspect. The yin channel will be more affected by cold because it is already naturally cold. The reproductive system and all of our organs are in front of the body and lie on the side of the Ren channel such as the stomach and the liver. This explains why all of them will be affected by the invasion of the liver channel by cold and all of them will pay the price and this price will affect their function aspect from an energetic, oriental, structural, anatomical and physiology perspective. For example, invasion of the kidney channel by cold will lead to kidney yang deficiency and to weakness in all of the back and spine especially the lower back and will also lead to frequent urination and the urine will be pale and colourless. The stomach channel can also be affected by the cold and in this case, the person will have rumbling and rattling noises in the stomach and bowel. We advise people with this condition to avoid anything below room temperature and to drink a lot of warm drinks and eat a lot of ginger and hot spicy food which will help to improve their condition. We also advise them to use a hot water bottle on the lower back, abdomen and lungs. When cold invades the spleen channel it leads to spleen yang deficiency which will affect the physical energy in general and the muscular strength also. It will also affect the digestive process in the stomach. Generally speaking, cold and yang deficiency is both what makes women's period much heavier in addition to physical exhaustion.

Liver Blood Deficiency

This condition is caused by a deficiency of Liver Blood. Many conditions lead to Liver blood deficiency. The main reasons for Liver blood deficiency are:

1. Haemorrhage – bleeding for a long period regardless of the cause for the bleeding, for example bleeding due to a trauma or a wound that has not healed. In these instances, the body will lose blood at a rapid rate which will affect the Livers capacity of storing the blood. Functions of the Liver include storing the blood and ensuring the smooth flow of qi when it is required. Qi and Blood will work together to ensure the release of the Blood to the working muscles, joints or ligaments. Qi and Blood are hugely linked and connected to all of our body functions continuously. Blood nourishes qi, qi pushes blood and blood cools and moistens the body's tissues and organs. When a huge quantity of blood is lost over a short period or if it lost due to a chronic disease or illness this will lead to anaemia from a western perspective. This is because there is not enough blood to nourish the qi and eventually qi becomes deficient and its movement slows and becomes stagnant and stops moving altogether.

2. Menstrual Cycle – If a woman has a heavy period or she bleeds more during than once during the menstruation cycle this will cause Liver blood deficiency and will also affect the woman's emotional state and the state of her health and well-being in general.

3. From a western perspective, there can be different reasons and causes for Liver blood deficiency including bleeding during a bowel motion and the bowel habit alternates between diarrhoea and constipation. These signs could also be indicative of the development of cancer particularly in the bowel however it does not mean we should jump to conclusions as there are accompanying signs to look out for such as rapid weight loss or loss of appetite and in severe cases vomiting after eating or drinking. When the tumour becomes advanced the person might alternate between feeling hot and feeling cold. Sometimes excessive bleeding from the bowel can also be due to Haemorrhoids especially in women. Haemorrhoids can appear during pregnancy and menstruation, particularly when the vascular system is put under pressure because the heart has to work harder to supply the blood, oxygen, nutrients and fluid to the growing foetus and the heart also has to cope with the fluctuations and the changes that take place in a women's body during pregnancy. A woman's blood pressure often fluctuates from being too low to too high during pregnancy. However, the blood pressure should be higher because the blood has to be pushed around the body and the circulation is intensified. The reason for this is related to the following theory whether from an oriental or a western perspective:

The formation of a new human being inside the woman's body is like a shock to the body especially if it is the first pregnancy for the woman. The woman's body needs a chance and time to adapt and accept the formation of the foetus in the body. At the start of the pregnancy the woman's body regards the foetus as having a foreign object in the body, this is despite the woman's body being designed and able to carry the task of conception and pregnancy from a physical aspect and an anatomy and physiology perspective.

However, the woman's body needs time to cope with the emotional changes Emotional attachment will be passed through the umbilical cord which carries everything to the foetus for it to grow and to develop. The woman eats, drinks, breathes and fights infection and disease for the baby during the pregnancy. During the first trimester of the pregnancy, the foetus is growing but will be closer to the upper portion of the body and so will be closer to the digestive, respiratory and vascular systems from a western perspective.

a) Because the foetus is closer to the stomach and lungs during the first trimester this will cause the woman to have morning sickness. This is because the pressure on the stomach makes the stomach acid moves upwards. From an oriental perspective, this is regarded as rebellious qi. If the woman vomits a lot during the first trimester it means a healthy pregnancy and baby as the toxins are being released.

b) The woman's breathing will become more shallow and faster because the foetus is close to the lungs and the proximity decreases the lungs shape and size and in return will decrease the lungs capacity for air oxygen intake hence the breathing becomes shallow and fast. Shallow and fast breathing will allow and make the blood pressure fluctuate especially making the blood pressure go higher. From a western perspective, the woman will have pre-eclampsia.

c) The heart beats faster and pumps blood faster to supply everything to the foetus through the umbilical cord, hence the blood pressure goes higher during this time. The pericardium is the muscular sac surrounding the heart and stored all our emotions which are carried through the umbilical cord to the foetus and from the foetus to the mother. Because of this connection through the umbilical cord, the fluctuation of the mother's emotions during the pregnancy will affect the foetus and from an oriental perspective the emotional state of the mother will become part of the new-born baby's physical make up in general. The best example to give is the lungs are related to sadness and grief and control the skin, if the mother has a lot of sadness and grief during the pregnancy this will make the baby more likely to be born with asthma, eczema or psoriasis or be more susceptible to have asthma, eczema or psoriasis later on in life.

d) During the last stage of pregnancy, the foetus will descend downwards hence the pressure will be no longer on the stomach and the lungs and the vomiting and morning sickness will have stopped, instead, the pressure is now on the kidneys, bladder, small intestine and large intestine. During this stage, the woman will have frequent urination, lower back pain, lack of physical strength and lack of energy in general because the baby is getting bigger and so the woman will be getting heavier. The foetus will put pressure on the bladder and the bowels and will decrease their size and shape which leads to the frequent urination and also to alternations between the bowel movements. However, constipation will be more predominant and sometimes will be accompanied by haemorrhoids which indicate a weakness in Spleen qi and Kidney qi especially kidney yang deficiency and spleen yang deficiency.

If the woman bleeds a lot during labour this can also lead to Liver Blood Deficiency. If the woman is anaemic before becoming pregnant or during pregnancy this will make matters worse. In severe cases, the woman needs a blood transfusion to help the situation.

Generally speaking, Liver Blood Deficiency shows the following signs and symptoms:

1. Dizziness and Disorientation

This is because there is not enough blood going to the head. Blood carries oxygen and when there is not enough blood there is not enough oxygen reaching the brain. The blood carries oxygen to all of the body organs and systems. The blood also carries glucose to support the body's functions, especially the brain. If the brain does not receive enough oxygen or glucose it will lead to a lack of memory, weakness, coma, fainting and death. People who have diabetes will faint when they do not enough insulin because they are not receiving enough glucose and this leads to fainting, weakness or coma. If they continue to not get insulin death will follow because all of the brains functions are affected.

2. Dryness

Dryness in all of the body will occur but particularly in the eyes because the liver opens into the eyes. The function of the blood is to cool and moisten all of the tissues and organs and also to nourish our senses. When there is a liver blood deficiency there will be no cooling and moistening for the eyes hence the eyes will be red, itchy, irritated and dry and in return, this will affect the sense of the sight. In general, the person will have blurred vision or weakness in the eyesight. In severe cases, the person will have a detached retina. If the person has liver blood deficiency with kidney yin deficiency they might start to develop cataracts in their eyes because the kidneys represent the old stage in life. Cataracts are part of the build-up of the ageing process over the years.

The following advice is recommended for people with liver blood deficiency:

➢ Stop the bleeding which causes the deficiency from the first place and ask the person to eat plenty of green vegetables with vitamin C which helps the absorption of the iron.

➢ Eat red meat with no fat in it no more than twice a week. The portion size each time should be half the palm of your hand.

➢ Eat vitamin A and vitamin D such as carrots and apples to improve their vision and eyesight in general.

➢ Chop an onion and put it in the bowl, cover your head with a towel and inhale the fumes of the onion until the eyes start tearing This will open the sinus and the tear duct and get rid of the dryness and will cool and moisten the eyes.

➢ Practice an exercise for the eyes to help the tear duct open and to prevent the dryness. The following exercise is recommended: Sit with your back straight and open your eyes as wide as you can. Stretch your lips, especially the top lip, as wide as you can and pick any point to gaze at. If you are sitting the point should be directly in front of you and if you are lying the point should be directly above you. Gaze at the point without blinking or frowning and you will feel the eyes start to get itchy and start to tear. Sometimes you will find that the tears are running more from one eye than the other. This indicates the blockage of the tear duct and the sinus from a western perspective and the stagnation of qi and blood, especially liver qi with blood and yin deficiency, from an oriental perspective. If the left eye is affected this means the yang aspect of the human body is more predominant. As we mentioned earlier the heart is a yin organ with a yang job to do which is circulate the blood, the blood is yin, but the movement of the blood is yang. This means you might not have the liver blood or liver yin deficiency, but you still have the eyesight problem like weakness of the sight or blurred vision. In this case, there is not enough yang qi to push the blood up to the eyes to cool and moisten the eyes to prevent the dryness and the blurred vision.

3. Pale Complexion

The person will look pale because there is not enough blood. There is not enough red blood cells to carry oxygen around the body up to the skin level hence the person and sometimes they will have dry skin and dry hair which falls out easily when brushed. The person will also have very weak and brittle hair and nails, especially the nails which will crack and break easily especially from a female aspect. From a western perspective, this is related to the deficiency of nutrients in the body, particularly vitamins. If a male if affected it will be related to their diet on one hand and the other hand it will be related to their testosterone level which is why men will have either impotence or premature ejaculation or premature greying of the hair and baldness of the hair.

4. Stiffness, Cramps and Spasms

The liver controls the sinews, the ligaments, cartilage and tendons, and so if liver blood is deficient this will lead to stiffness, cramps and spasms making it difficult to move with agility and flexibility. Any simple and basic movement becomes an effort and a struggle. The reason for this is because there will not be enough blood to give the sinews the agility and elasticity to perform the movement freely and smoothly. One of the functions of the liver is to ensure the smooth flow of qi, all of our body parts and organs are connected like a jigsaw, therefore tightness and stiffness of the sinews leads to tightness and stiffness of the joint and the muscles which will lead to spasm and cramps. It is like a vicious because when the sinews are not free the joint is not allowed to move and when the joint is stiff it doesn't allow the muscle to move and this circle keep ongoing. The human body is not designed to stay still and the best advice is to improve the flexibility of the sinews, muscles and joints and to keep them active all of the time by doing stretching and exercises and join either yoga or Pilates class. Swimming and cycling, especially on an indoor exercise bike, will also help the sinews, muscles and joints regain the flexibility and mobility that the person needs to carry out their daily activities and ordinary work. If you do not know how to swim just holding onto the rail in the swimming pool and moving your joint while the body is floating in the water will help you sinews, joints and muscles. It is important when using an exercise bike that you cycle the correct way, by this I mean cycle with your feet completely straight without turning your toes in or your heels out, your small toe should be level and parallel with your heel and your heel should be level with your shoulder. The same principle applies when you walk, people who walk with their toes out sometimes end up having a knee replacement and people who walk with their toes turned in sometimes end up having a hip replacement. If you look at your shoes you will be able to see where they are wearing from. If they are wearing from the big toe to the arch the person may have a knee replacement if the shoe is wearing from the small toes to the heel the person may have a hip replacement because the same process that is happening to the shoes is also happening internally in the joint. This indicates the importance of posture in general whether you are standing, sitting, jogging, walking, static or moving. The spine should be completely straight and when you look forward your neck should not be tilted right or left and your nose should be between your two big toes. From an anatomical and physiology perspective, this indicates that your spine is straight.

5. Numbness of the Limbs

Liver blood deficiency leads to an emptiness in the vessels and in the channels this emptiness will be filled by a mild version of internal wind which will create spasm and numbness. This numbness will be felt along the pathway of the channel and its connected structure. The wind is yang in nature and yang rises upwards towards the face and head hence the person will have dry and twitchy eyes, blurred vision and dizziness. When this wind reaches the head it will affect the equilibrium pressure the ear, face and head and sometimes this dizziness will be there all of the time or sometimes it will only be there with a certain movement that the person does especially sudden and jerking movements such as when the person is cycling or turning from side to side

6. Abnormal Menstrual Cycle

The woman might have a very light and scanty period or they might have a very long and heavy period. This will depend on the amount of wind which fills the vessels and will depend on the deficiency of the liver yin and the stagnation of liver qi. The best way to describe it is like a tap of water and the water comes from the tap too fast or the water only comes in drops.

This is because of the exhaustion of liver blood and liver qi which is not able to push and ensure the smooth flow of qi. This will lead not only to the stagnation of blood and qi but also to the emotional stagnation of liver qi. The main emotion linked and connected to the liver is anger, hatred, resentment, frustration and jealousy which strongly affects the woman's emotional feelings all of the time but especially either before or after their period or during the ovulation time. From a western perspective, this indicates the hormonal imbalance between the progesterone, which is yang in nature and has the function to warm up and push out and start the period, and the oestrogen, which is yin in nature and has the function to cool and moisten and prepare the body for fertility and conception. These two hormones, progesterone and oestrogen, will influence the woman's health and wellbeing in general almost all of the time.

Liver Wind turning into Heat

This condition is caused by the invasion of the heat which comes from the exterior environment and settles in the interior environment. The wind tends to invade the liver as an organ and as a channel before invading any other organ or channel. This explains why the liver is hugely and directly linked to any condition which is related to wind, shakes, convulsions, tics, tremors, moving, jumping and jerking from an oriental perspective. From a western perspective, this condition is related to the neurological system and also to the immune system.

1) Wind makes the tree branches shake

Our extremities are similar to the branches of the tree, especially in the arms. A person with Parkinson's disease or epilepsy will have shaking and quivering moments because when the wind heat goes down to the interior and demolishes and damages liver blood and burns up liver yin. In return, this will cause massive heat n the body and over long periods the heat will turn into internal wind which causes the internal shaking and quivering of the extremities.

2) High Fever and High Temperature

This is because wind and heat are both yang in nature. Yang is a form of heat and yang rises however in this case it is a very extreme form of heat which turns into fire. For example, if you put your finger into hot water you will feel the heat from the water that burns your finger, but if you immediately put your finger on the fire you will feel the heat also but it is a different form of heat than the kind you felt when you put your finger in the water.

3) Red and dry face. Sometimes only the cheeks will be red.

4) Bloodshot eyes or in severe cases, bleedings from the eyes.

This liver fire can be so intense that rises into the head and the eyes. If the persons' ankles are twisted this will affect this sight as a sense and the eyes and also the hearing as a sense and the ears and sometimes may lead to migraines and vertigo. A twisted ankle will cause the vision and the hearing on the same side to pay price.

5)   Bleeding from the eyes or nose or both.

This is caused by intense liver fire and wind which puts a huge amount of pressure on the anterior wall of the arteries and capillaries. When these arteries and capillaries are not able to cope with this pressure they start to rupture. The capillaries are so small in size and shape that they are not able to cope with this pressure. The consequences of this will be either bleeding from the eyes, nose or both. This can be a common occurrence in children who have a habit of picking their nose or it can also happen when there is a direct blow to the nose or eyes but especially the nose, or when the weather is hot and humid and the intensity of the heat will cause the bleeding particularly from the nose.

6)   Bitter taste or bitter and sour taste in the mouth and throat. This is caused by hyperactivity of the liver fire and liver wind at the same time.

7)   Feeling angry and frustrated.

The person becomes angry, frustrated and upset very easily. This is because anger is the emotion linked and connected to the liver as an organ and the liver as a channel. Each structure that the liver channel passes through from start to finish will be affected and will pay the price for this anger. Generally speaking, anger, resentment, frustration, hatred and jealousy which are generated by liver fire and liver wind will lead stiffness, cramps, spasms and tightness. The muscles become very tense and hard to the touch. This is because the liver controls the sinews which become tight and rigid and will shrink in size and shape which will, in turn, affect the flexibility of the joint and muscles and movement will be difficult. Every moment will become difficult to do regardless of whether the person is sitting, standing, resting or moving. Sometimes these symptoms can be worse at night when the person is lying in bed and they will find it difficult to find a comfortable position to lie in and will keep twisting and turning. To encourage a peaceful nights sleep it is recommended to do the following:

➢ Don't go to bed with a full stomach

➢ It's important to"wind down" before going to bed by meditating, praying or by hypnosis.

➢ Deep and slow breathing is essential for the process to take place

➢ Drink a lot of water throughout the day especially first thing in the morning to wash the body's systems and organs from the acidity and toxins that go through it during the day. The more neutralised and alkaline the body is and toxin-free the better the body will function and the easier the sleeping process will be.

➢ Contemplation and visualisation that you are in the sleeping stage even before going to bed helps also

➢ Chanting a spiritual prayer, especially silently, with yourself allows you to your subconscious which is very important for the sleeping process to take place from start to finish.

➢ Avoid watching violent films before bed as these will create hyperactivity

➢ If you find it difficult to visualise, contemplate or hypnotise yourself your practitioner will be able to give you a programmer designed for you as an individual to practice at home to help you to have a peaceful night's sleep.

8) The tongue coating will be yellow because the heat has accumulated and turns into damp heat.

9) The pulse will be very wiry and rapid because heat and wind together cause hyperactivity hence the fast and rapid pulse.

What I mean when I say the condition is formed by a very extreme form of heat which turns to wind and which is then circulated internally and moves with the circulation of the blood.

The signs and symptoms that will be produced when the liver wind turns into the fire will be far more serious for the person as they are regarded as life-threatening signs whether looked at from an oriental medical perspective or western medical perspective.

➢ Generally speaking, any high temperature is a sign that indicates the seriousness of the condition.

➢ Fire and wind both will become the main cause for the high temperature. If the temperature continues to rise the heat and wind will also rise and cause convulsions. The best example of thus us meningitis which is an inflammation of the meningeal layer that covers the brain and is caused by a bacterial infection. It is a very serious and deadly condition. A person with meningitis will have a very rigid and stiff back of the neck. The reason for this from an oriental perspective is because the Du channel, which is on the back of the spine, represents the heat and yang aspect of the human body, its opposite yin channel is the Ren which is on the front of the body and represents the yin and cooling and moistening aspect of the human body. The invasion of the Du channel by liver wind and the liver fire causes the person to have a stiff and rigid neck. Because the channel itself is already related to heat this liver wind and liver fire will be like adding petrol to the fire when it invades any channel but especially the Du channel which has the heating function and aspect from an oriental perspective. If you want to look at it from a western perspective you will find that the same reasons cause the convulsions, shaking, stiffness and rigidity of the neck. The reason for this is because the hypothalamus lies in the base of the skull on the back of the neck and has the function of acting like a human thermostat similar to what you would have at home in your heating system that adjusts itself automatically according to the external temperature. The invasion of the hypothalamus in regulating body temperature. This means the temperature only has the potential of rising and not going down to its normal degree. This will be another reason for the convulsions because at this stage the wind and heat are gone down to cellular level and in the blood and will be circulated by the heart to all the body's systems and organ especially the extremities and the brain because the brain needs a huge amount of blood, oxygen and fluid to be in control of all body functions.

➢ The liver opens into the eyes and the wind fire will invade the eyes and make them stare upward and the person will no longer be able to control their eye movement. In very severe cases this will lead to fainting, coma and even death of the affected person. The main reason for fainting and coma is because the liver wind and liver fire will invade the pericardium, the muscular sac surrounding the heart where we carry all of our emotions since the day we were born and before we were born, and when this happens the person's mind will be affected. This is because the pericardium is part of the heart and is linked and connected to the heart as an organ and as a channel and one of the functions of the heart from an oriental perspective is to capture the mind. When this liver wind and heat enters the pericardium the heart will be no longer able to capture the mind because of the damage and destruction that the liver wind and fire cause to the heart yin and the pericardium yin. Subsequently, the mind will not be captured and when the mind is lost the condition starts to go from bad to worse, from the mind not being captured into disorientation being disturbed, hysteria and delirium and this will eventually cause the person to faint and go into a coma and death will follow.

➤ Because the wind and heat have gone to blood level and are being circulated throughout our body down to a cellular level the person will have a very red face and very red tongue, especially the tip of the tongue, along with a very fast and rapid pulse. The reason for this is because the wind and heat cause hyperactivity which makes the heart beat faster and in return makes the person have very dangerously high blood pressure. Four examples from western medicine that relate wind fire are Meningitis, Epilepsy, Parkinson's, Bell's Palsy.

Meningitis: This is an inflammation of the brain layer and is caused by a bacterial infection which has already been discussed above.

Epilepsy: This is not a disease which passes from person to person. Epilepsy is an indication that tells us that there is something wrong with part of the brain structure which affects the function of the brain. From an oriental perspective, epilepsy is defined as the dysfunctional aspect of the liver which is responsible for making live qi and liver blood to flow freely and smoothly. From a western perspective, the same theory is applied when we talk about epilepsy, it is defined as the disturbance of the output and the flow of the electric signals that are generated by the brain. The best way to describe this is an electrical sign that is generated by the brain is like an electrical wire that receives huge amounts of electrical volts that the wire is not able to deal and cope with. The same thing will happen to the body during an epileptic fit because these electrical signals come suddenly and compulsively and in vast volumes. This gives the body, brain and heart a massive shock which will lead to cramps, spasm, contraction and stiffness of the muscles which make the neck go rigid and tight, makes the limbs weak, the breathing difficult and the speech incoherent. This will affect all of the body's functions including memory, which is why many with epilepsy don't recollect what happened. The stronger the fit and the stronger the signs and symptoms are, the stronger the impact and effect on the health of the affected person.

Parkinson's: Parkinson's is a chronic progressive and slow disease. When a person has Parkinson's, their brain will be affected. This means there is a disturbance of the functions of the small centre of the brain. The person will have:

a) Tremor and shaking of the extremities the arms and hands. In return, this will affect the person's grip and balance when they try to pick up or hold any object using either one hand or both.

b) Stiffness and tightness of the muscles and joints which leads to difficulty when the person is moving. All movement becomes slow and difficult.

Bell's Palsy: This is paralysis of the facial nerve. Sometimes it is only temporary for a short period and sometimes it is a longer period and is chronic. When a person has Bell's Palsy, they will not be able to use their facial muscles and the muscles of the mouth and eyes hence they are dropped to one side and will lead to an inability for the person to speaks. Sometimes the vision in both eyes will be affected and sometimes only the eye on the affected side will be affected. The affected eye will become runny and foggy. The muscles of the forehead will also be affected by the loss of feeling and sensation and hence the person will not be able to frown or close their eyes.

To make the idea of wind-heat or wind-cold easy to understand will take epilepsy as an example. Epilepsy is regarded as a condition which is caused by the invasion of wind internally. Liver wind invades all of the body in general but especially the pericardium as a channel and the pericardium as a muscular sac surrounding the heart. This sac is filled with fluid which is regarded as yin and which has the function to cool and moisture from an oriental perspective and has the function of preventing friction between the heart and its surrounding structures from a western perspective. When the wind settles in the internal environment of our body it will affect the blood flow, heart rhythm, brain activities and brain signals hence the epileptic fit takes place because this wind has gone internal. The wind passes the Wei qi which is our defensive qi and represents our immune system from a western perspective and represents our skin and muscular system from an oriental perspective. After passing through the Wei Qi this wind goes further down to nutritive qi which is equivalent to the interstitial fluid that our cells swim in. the wind then goes down to blood level and starts to interfere with all of the body's systems and organs but it especially interferes with the blood, which is regarded as an organ from an oriental perspective, and with the heart because the heart has to circulate the blood and also interferes with the brain, all of which causes the epileptic fit.

If we compare epilepsy with Bell's Palsy both conditions are caused by the invasion of wind-heat, but with Bell's Palsy, the wind is caused by the external invasion, for example driving the car with only one window open or being exposed to very cold and windy weather. The wind and cold will invade the facial muscles and all of the channels they pass through but if this wind goes down to blood level it will turn to heat and will start to dry and demolish the yin. Wind heat is more serious and damaging to our health than the wind cold. From an oriental perspective when someone has an invasion of wind-cold it matches the saying 'caught in a draught' where someone has a stiff/tight neck as a result of a draught blowing on it. Generally speaking, the wind-heat and fire is a more serious and life-threatening condition than wind-cold when it comes to the treatment of the condition whether looked at from an oriental perspective or a western perspective. For example, meningitis is more life-threatening hat bell's Palsy. Regardless of what condition the person has the job of the practitioner is to create the balance and that's what our medicine is all about, creating the balance between yin and yang.

CHAPTER 5

THE FUNCTIONS OF THE HEART

The heart from a western perspective acts as a pump, circulating the blood around all the body systems and tissues and organs. However, from an oriental perspective when we talk about the heart, we do not talk from an anatomy physiology perspective, such as the heart has a left and right atrium or ventricle or the valves to regulate the blood flow. Instead, we talk about the six functions which are completely unrelated to the western perspective.

1) Controls channel and blood vessels

The heart controls the channels and blood vessels, which means circulation. The channels and blood vessels represent the veins and arteries and capillaries.

Veins are muscular tubes. They carry deoxygenated blood. Arteries are also muscular tubes. They carry oxygenated blood. Capillaries are the smallest of the body's blood vessels. They cover every part of the body. There are nerve capillaries and blood capillaries which carry nutrients and oxygen and sensation to every part of our body.

The left side of the body represents the yang aspect. Yang is the activity, movement, it warms the body. Yang is equivalent to progesterone from a female aspect and testosterone from a male aspect. The heart is a yin organ with a yang job to do. Yin is dense, material, substantial and tangible. The yin organ has to work 24 hours a day and so the heart circulates 24 hours a day. The small intestine is the hearts paired organ, which is a yang organ.

Blood comes from the left side of the heart. This is oxygenated blood. This is why varicose veins are generally worse on the right side of the body because the body is going up against gravity – back up to the heart again. The spleen represents the functional aspect of the heart from an oriental perspective. The spleen has to push the Qi, hold the qi and hold the organ upwards for 24 hours a day. It also has to hold the blood and fluids in place, because the blood is regarded as an organ from an oriental perspective. If there is any leakage of blood or fluid, especially in the lower extremities and in particular around the ankle, calf or knee means that the spleen is not holding blood in place. If we feel tired we normally feel it in our legs but especially the calve muscles that's because the spleen circulates against gravity.

To link a western perspective between the spleen and heart from an oriental perspective I will give you the following example: if a person has a clot due to circulatory problem in most cases the clot forms in the lower leg below the knee and especially in the calve muscles. In this case, because the spleen represents the functional aspect of the heart and the heart has to circulate the deoxygenated blood back to the lungs that explain why in most cases the cloth will travel from the calve to the lungs.

The circulation in the vascular system from a western perspective represented by the circulation of qi and blood from an oriental perspective. As we said earlier blood nourishes qi and qi has to push the blood in the channels and blood vessels and this represents the circulation from an oriental perspective. The interaction between qi and blood will form the quality of the pulse that the human has. The quality and type of pulse will be affected and determined by a number of factors.

The pulse is affected by the way you eat when you eat and what you eat. Most of the digestion process takes place in the small intestine. The digestion process starts from the first second you put the food into your mouth. Chewing the food for a long enough period allows the saliva in the mouth to work with the enzymes to aid the digestion process and to decrease the amount of work the stomach has to do and the amount of gastric juices the stomach needs for digestion.

You have probably heard at some stage that it is not recommended to eat while you are standing or moving around. The reason for this is because you are damaging your stomach as an organ and undermining the spleen as a function and symptoms such as indigestion, belching, burping or heartburn may occur. The spleen is a yin organ and its paired yang organ is the stomach. The spleen has to extract the nutrients from the food you eat. When you eat standing up you are interfering with the circulation and digestion at the same time. Also, when you eat or drink straight from the fridge it will affect the circulation from a western perspective and it will undermine the spleen from an oriental perspective. As we mentioned, daytime is yang and night-time is yin. The yin is equivalent to the gastric juices and endorphins (natural painkillers) and the serotonin. It is not good to eat two or three hours before bedtime because you demolish your yin in general but especially the stomach yin which is equivalent to the gastric juices. When you want to go to sleep the parasympathetic and the subconscious are in charge of the sleeping process. When you eat your brain and the sympathetic nervous system is in charge of the digestion process. In this case, when you eat two to three hours before bedtime you are creating a huge conflict between the sympathetic system and the parasympathetic system and between the brain and mind and the subconscious. Eating too close to bedtime, especially a large meal, too much red meat, too much carbohydrate or too much oily greasy food will result in a conflict taking place in your body and also your mind. The reason for this is because the circulation goes down to the stomach to start the digestive system instead of going up to the brain and the subconscious to start the sleeping process. This conflict between the physical body, which is represented by the digestive system as a system and the stomach as an organ, and the mind and subconscious, which is regarded as an organ from an oriental perspective albeit a non-physical, non-tangible and non-substantial organ, will lead to the following symptoms when you go to bed: indigestion, burping, belching, heartburn, hiccups, wind, difficulty finding a comfortable position in bed and either not being able to fall asleep in the first place or if you do fall asleep, not being able it maintain a peaceful nights sleep. When you wake during the night most of your thinking will be negative and you will be expecting the worst scenario and creating your delusional image asking yourself why, when or how questions without being able to find an answer. Each time you eat the pancreas produce insulin to control the amount of sugar in the blood. The pancreas from a western perspective represents the spleen from an oriental perspective. This relation makes sense as the spleen controls the sweet taste. From an anatomy and physiology perspective, the spleen is on the left side of the body and is opposite to the gallbladder, which is on the right side of the body. Each time you eat the gallbladder has to produce bile to burn the fat. Bile is a form of liquid. The bile and insulin combine and move towards the stomach and will explain why indigestion and symptoms mentioned above occur.

From an oriental perspective, the world is built on yin and yang and the five elements. This is from every aspect including from a nutritional aspect. For a meal to be balanced and healthy it should contain the five elements:

1) *Carbohydrates*

Excess carbohydrate means there is too much sugar which leads to diabetes and in return will affect the circulation. You will often see people with diabetes also having poor circulation, especially in the lower limbs and the feet and in the big toe. Too little carbohydrate means there is not enough sugar in the body and can result in hypoglycaemia causing tiredness, lethargy and weakness. Over a long period this weakness cold cause a person to faint.

From an oriental perspective, we always say that deficiency is better than excess. This is because the deficiency is something you could add to. It is very easy to add something to the body however it is very difficult to expel excess from the body. Excess is something that should not be in there in the first place. Examples include:

• Diarrhoea, a deficiency condition which is preferable to constipation, an excess condition. With diarrhoea the body can expel the toxins however with constipation the toxins are building and over a long period could lead to cancer.

- Heavy periods, a deficiency condition, which is preferable to having no period, an excess condition.

- Anaemia (too little iron) is preferable to Hemochromatosis (too much iron) which is regarded as an excess. It is very difficult to expel excess iron from the body.

- Low blood pressure is deficiency and is generally regarded as safer than high blood pressure which is regarded as an excess regardless of the cause. High blood pressure over a long period could lead to a stroke which could lead to paralysis. There are two types of stroke, a yin stroke and a yang stroke. The yin stroke occurs when a clot is formed in the blood and travels to the brain and blocks the vein, artery or capillary. The outcome will depend on where the stroke takes place in the brain and what part of the brain is affected. If the stroke occurs in the part of the brain which controls body movements, the body movements and the balance will be affected. If the stroke were to occur in the part of the brain related to speech. The yang stroke from a western perspective is known as an aneurysm. this occurs when the vein, artery or capillary in the brain either leak or rupture. From an oriental perspective, this is related to the spleen. The spleen from an oriental perspective represents the heart from a western perspective. From an oriental perspective, the spleen also has the function of holding the organs in place and the blood is regarded as an organ. Generally speaking, this type of stroke is more difficult to treat. The treatment plan should include moving the blood away from the affected side, trying to make the client bleed or increasing the amount of blood in a woman's period. The treatment plan outlined above mentions increasing the amount of blood in a woman's period. Any medical condition is easier to treat in a female because the woman can be treated through the period and also at the time of ovulation. Observing the tongue and the pulse at these times helps the practitioner to decide whether the period needs to be increased or decreased. From an oriental perspective, women are viewed as having a longer life span than men. This is because women have the monthly menstruation and ovulation process which is seen as a purification and filtering process. The process can be compared to the oil in a car, if you do not change the oil it will become dirty and will affect the function of the car. In this case, the oil is the blood. When the woman bleeds it forces the bone marri to re-generate and make new blood cells. Men could consider donating blood to obtain a similar purification process.

2) Protein

Consuming too much protein can result in calcifications and any form of bunions. Generally speaking, protein accumulates in the circulation and circulates all around the body. This accumulation of protein mainly affects the lower limbs and the foot, particularly the big toe where the spleen channel starts. As was mentioned earlier, the spleen from an oriental perspective represents the heart and circulation from a western perspective. Not consuming enough protein results in a lack of energy, even when you are doing nothing.

3) Fat

Too much fat leads to cholesterol which blocks the veins and arteries and as a result makes the hearts job of pushing the blood through the veins, arteries and capillaries much more difficult. This puts a massive amount of pressure on the anterior wall of these vessels which leads to high blood pressure. High blood pressure can be defined as the amount of pressure the blood puts upon the anterior wall of the veins, arteries and capillaries when it flows through them. This pressure depends on what you eat, your weight, your lifestyle in general and your feelings.

Not enough fat in your body will lead to the decline and decrease of the mental capacity including your memory, both short term and long term, your focus and your concentration and intellect. This is because the body in general cannot function without fat. There is a certain area in our brain that cannot function without fat which is why fish oils are beneficial and also eating plenty of fresh fish.

4) Vitamins

Vitamins are very important in the diet. Eating six pieces of fruit a day is very beneficial to get all the required vitamins. Eating two pieces with each meal is a good way to make it a habit. However, it is important not to eat fruit on an empty stomach except for apple. Apple is alkaline and neutralises the acid in the stomach. Our body does not store vitamins which is why we need a continuous supply regularly in our food. During the night the stomach produces acid to prepare for the digestion process the following day. Eating fruit (except the apple) on an empty stomach in the morning adds acid to the already existing acid. Many people visit an acupuncturist complaining of digestive problems and stomach problems including Crohn's disease and ulcerative colitis. These people will usually say that their symptoms worsen after eating too much fruit without keeping the diet balance that we are currently discussing. By eating a lot of fruit you are abusing your gastric juices which are produced by the stomach and you are also abusing you gastric enzymes which are along all your digestive tract. The digestion process begins with chewing food in the mouth. The gastric enzymes are triggered when you chew the food which commences the digestive process. The more gastric enzymes you have the better your digestion will be. People who smoke don't have a good sense of taste, this is because their enzymes in the saliva are either destroyed or damaged which in turn affects their sense of taste and also their sense of smell and subsequently affects their appetite in general. When people quit up smoking they can see a change in their weight.

The body can regenerate itself down to a cellular level. This means everything in the digestive tract will be renewed. When a person gives up smoking he body regenerates itself and the person will look fresher, younger and healthier. The taste buds and smell sense cells will also regenerate new cells resulting in a stronger sense of taste and smell. This will then improve the appetite and the digestive system in general. Acupuncture can help with giving up smoking and managing weight gain. There are specific acupuncture points which, when used, tell the brain to decide what the person needs according to their physical activity. This means the brain will decide on the number of calories the person needs. When we feel hungry a message goes from the brain to the stomach and we start to eat. When we feel full a message goes back from the stomach to the brain and we stop eating, this can be applied to any physical process in the body such as the kidneys, bladder and bowel.

There are a variety of vitamins such as vitamin A, vitamin C, vitamin K or vitamin D along with many more. Each vitamin has its purpose and function in the body. For example, the function of vitamin C s to support the immune system and to fight infection.

The purpose of vitamin D is to support bones. Vitamin A is related to the sight and vitamin K is related to the process of coagulation.

5) *Water*

Seventy per cent of the body is water. A human could live for a month without food however the body cannot survive without water, after three days the body starts to die because the cells start to float. The best form of water is the kind which does not contain any fluoride or chloride such as the filtered water.

The brain is muscular and jelly-like and the spinal column, which is linked to the brain, is filled with the cerebral spinal fluid. This fluid is from water, jelly-like and has a white colour. When testing for meningitis doctors will carry out a lumbar puncture on lumbar 4 and will remove some fluid for examinations. If the fluid is blue, it means the person has meningitis. Another characteristic of meningitis is a red rash that does not disappear when you press a glass on it. The reason for choosing lumber 4 is because it is anarea which is rich in nerve endings. Lumber 4 is also used when giving an epidural. This area where lumbar 4 is situated represents the kidneys from an oriental perspective. From an oriental perspective, the stomach represents life. When in the womb the foetus is connected to the mother through the umbilical cord which is through the stomach. Through the umbilical cord, everything is done by the mother for the baby such as eating, breathing and fighting infections. This is why it represents life. From an oriental perspective lumbar 4 represents death and is known as the Gate of Vitality. Generally speaking, if you drink large amounts of fluid you should also take salt to keep the balance. When a person drinks too much water in a short period the kidneys cannot flush it out fast enough and the blood becomes waterlogged. Water enters the body when we drink and is removed primarily in the urine and sweat. Drinking to much water lowers the concentration of salt in the cells. Balancing the water intake with salt can help to overcome this problem by keeping the balance.

2) Manifests in the complexion

From an oriental perspective, the complexion manifests itself everywhere, not only in the face. However the fact, legs and extremities can reflect the state of the circulation. The complexion depends on the heats circulation and so the stronger the hearts circulation is, the better the complexion will be and vice versa.

The complexion can vary according to your emotional state and to your health in general.

If a person is happy and healthy the heart and circulation will work to their optimum level. This will show in all of the body but especially in the skin and the face. The face will be shiny, moist and glowing with rosy cheeks. This is a sign of strong circulation and healthy skin. The heart is related to joy, excitement and happiness and the lungs are related to sadness and grief. The lungs control the is and hair of the body and if you are sad, upset or in a state of grief this will affect your complexion which will show itself in the skin in general but especially in the face. When you are experiencing feelings of sadness or grief your breathing becomes shallow and weak resulting in your body and skin not receiving enough oxygen. Oxygen is carried in the blood which is pumped by the heart. The less amount of oxygen the skin receives the drier it will be which ultimately speeds up the ageing process. Wearing a lot of makeup on the skin will also affect the quality of the skin. The skin, like every other organ in the body, needs to breathe and needs oxygen. By putting on a lot of makeup this will decrease the amount of oxygen getting to the skin. Also, the chemicals existing in makeup can speed up the ageing process.

If you are in a state of shock the shock will suspend the energy from moving smoothly and freely. Shock is related to the kidneys from an oriental perspective. The function of the kidneys is to filter the blood which purifies and cleanses the blood. This in turn will impact the texture and tone of the skin and reduce the number of wrinkles and frown lines on the skin as the skin are receiving pure and cleansed blood which is full of oxygen. From a western perspective if a person has kidney failure they will inevitably also have heart failure and vice versa.

The emotion of anger will also reflect on the complexion. When we are angry, we tend to tense up and frown. The action of frowning will deplete and deprive the muscles, and in particular the facial muscles, from oxygen and nutrients because the tightening of the muscles restricts the movement and flow of the oxygen and nutrients. Frowning also affects our sense of judgement and perception because it affects our third eye, which is located between the eyebrows. The more the eyes are squinted the less the eyes and face will receive oxygen. This may lead to dry eyes and face and may weaken the eyesight. The Liver is related to anger, hatred, resentment and frustration and the liver opens into the eyes. The more anger you have the more you will frown or squint and your eyesight and complexion will be affected. If you to go an ophthalmologist, you will get a prescription for glasses. However, the stronger the glasses the weaker your eyesight will become because glasses are not designed to deal with anger or hatred. Strong glasses will also make you squint or frown and so it is a vicious circle.

3) Health in General

The complexion depends on your state of health and the state of your wellbeing in general. As I mentioned earlier, red blood cells are yin and they carry oxygen, white blood cells are yang and they carry lymph to fight infection. This explains why when you are sick you look pale and your skin will be dry. The reason for this is because the immune system and lymphatic system receive a message from the brain telling them to increase the white blood cells to fight the infection for the sick person. In this case, the white blood cells increase and outnumber the red blood cells and the person will look pale, dry and exhausted. From an oriental perspective, we talk about a pre-existing condition waiting for the trigger to start it. For example, two people are sitting in the same room and the next day one of them has the flu and a temperature and is sweating and shivering. From an oriental perspective they are both in the same environment and breathing the same air in the same room so why did one person get the flu and the other did not? This means, from an oriental perspective, the person who got the flu has either physical weakness or a weakness in the immune system and lymphatic system. This means the person had a pre-existing condition. When a person has these weaknesses they may refer to themselves as feeling 'run down'. Another example of having a pre-existing condition for a physical weakness can be seen if two people run at the same speed and hit the same wall. One of them will have bruises and the other will not. Hitting the wall triggered a condition and shows the reality of physical strength and physical constitution. The same applies from an emotional aspect. For example, the lungs are related to sadness and grief and two people may respond differently to the sadness as a trigger to their emotion.

4) Controls Sweating

From an oriental perspective, the heart controls sweating. Generally speaking, sweating is defined as a purification and cleansing process for all our body systems and organs. Sweating helps to regulate body temperature and sweating also helps the metabolic rate of the fluid and salt intake.

There is yin sweating and yang sweating. If you sweating during the daytime and you sweat a lot when you are active this is related to yang deficiency. If you sweat at night especially while you are at rest, sitting or sleeping, this is related to yin deficiency.

From an oriental perspective there are three types of sweating:

a) Sweating during physical activity

The heart beats between seventy and eight beats a minute while at rest. When you exercise the heart has to speed up and so the number of beats per minute increases. Sweat and activity is a form of yang and heat. When the heart circulates blood around the body, especially to the working muscles to sustain the action of exercising, this process will produce waste which is partly made up of uric and lactic acid. The body tries to protect itself from the build-up of toxins and uric and lactic acid through the process of sweating. This is a healthy form of sweating because the person is doing physical activity and they are doing cardiovascular actions which force the heart to pump and to circulate at a faster speed. This will also help to decrease the body fat and cholesterol level and will also help to increase the physical body's stamina, fitness and endurance.

b)   Sweating while at rest

Sweating without doing physical activity from an oriental perspective is one of the warning signs of physical weakness and also a weakness related to the immune system and lymphatic systems. This is regarded as an unhealthy form of sweating because the body is losing salt, fluid and nutrients for no specific reason.

The location of sweating from an oriental perspective will be determined what channel is involved and what organ is affected:

- Sweating from the armpit is related to the heart as an organ and also as a channel
- Sweating from the palm is related to the lungs and pericardium
- Sweating from the nose, especially while you are eating, is related to the spleen as a channel and as an organ.
- Sweating from the forehead, especially the hairline, is related to the stomach as a channel and as an organ.

Regardless of the channel affected and the organ involved sweating without physical activity is a sign of physical weakness from an oriental perspective, most likely a weakness related to the muscles and skin.

There are certain situations when sweating in a hot environment may be beneficial to you. People with high blood pressure, especially high blood pressure caused by overconsumption of salt, will benefit from going to a sauna and sweating in the sauna. This is because when they sweat they will sweat out the excess salt.

However, if a person has low blood pressure the opposite applies. Sweating in a hot environment such as a sauna will cause the person to sweat out salt which they don't have enough of in the first place. If the high blood pressure is caused by anger or physical exhaustion, such as lack of sleep, the sauna will not be a solution. The same can be applied to the sleeping process. Physical activity and tiredness will lead to exhaustion. If a lifestyle is hectic and they are not getting enough rest or sleep they will have exhaustion. If they change their lifestyle and get more rest and sleep then the physical exhaustion will be dealt with and helped with. Unfortunately, this cannot be applied to emotional issues. If a person is angry you cannot tell them to go to sleep and that they will feel better when they wake up and that the anger will be gone. The physical rest will deal with the external physical body but the emotional rest needs to go down to the cellular level. The difference between physical exhaustion and emotional exhaustion can be seen at times when you feel physically exhausted but your mind and subconscious are still able to function to its optimum and maximum level of alertness and concentration. The same could be applied to people which mental disabilities however physically their body could be stronger than someone else's.

There is a fourth type of sweating which is caused by the use of medications such as antibiotics or illegal drugs such as heroin or cocaine. Sweating is a process of purification and cleansing. When a person uses drugs this will put the body under a huge amount of pressure especially the skin, which is the largest organ in the human body, as it tries to expel as much toxin as it can to protect the person.

5) Makes Blood

The heart makes blood through the process of eating. When a person eats a well-balanced diet containing the five elements this means the body will be able to manufacture new red blood cells. These new red blood cells are manufactured in the thigh bone on the femur. This explains why if a person does not eat or they make themselves sick, as can be seen, is illnesses such as anorexia or bulimia. They will look pale as new red blood cells are not being created. If the new blood cells are created they will be deficient of nutrients. As we now know the heart controls the complexion and in the case of a person who does not eat, the heart is not receiving enough nutrients which will then affect the circulation in general. The red blood cells in our body are constantly being replaced by new red blood cells. The same applies to white blood cells. If the newborn cell is deprived of oxygen, nutrients and fluids there will be a pre-existing weakness. For example, if a pregnant woman does not eat well her baby will be undernourished and may be born underweight and in severe cases may not survive. In this case, the baby had a pre-existing weakness which had been inherited from the mother due to the mother not eating enough nutrients and therefore resulting in not enough blood being manufactured for the mother but especially for the baby. This explains why a well-balanced diet is very important for everyone.

6) Captures the Mind

From an oriental perspective, the mind is completely separate from the brain. The brain is physical, tangible and substantial but the activities such as memory, concentration, focus, intellect, mental capacity, wisdom, intuition and perception are non-physical, non-tangible and non-substantial. You can take an x-ray of the brain, see the brain, touch the brain but from a western perspective you cannot take an x-ray or scan of the mind. From an oriental perspective, however, we can take a non-physical x-ray of the mind. The mind is related to the subconscious and the parasympathetic nervous system. The mind controls your thoughts, behaviour and your way of thinking if you ask your friend do they know what you are thinking they will tell you they do not. This is what we mean, from an oriental perspective, about taking a non-physical x-ray or scan of the mind to access the internal subconscious state of the human being deep down to cellular level. From an oriental perspective, your emotions can be described as being like layers of an onion. Two people can carry the same emotion such as sadness or anger but the emotional state of each of them will be at a different cellular level and will have a different frequency and vibration which creates the reaction of the person according to the situation which is provoking them. For example, if two people are sad and one of them is sad for one week and the other is sad for ten years or since the day they were born, who will be at a deeper level of emotional state if compared to the onion? The answer is the person who has the sadness for ten years. As we mentioned earlier concerning sexual activity, the activity does not represent the structural aspect i.e. the penis, rectum or vagina, or the action of them. It represents the state of your mind and also the state of your emotional feelings and behaviour at the time. During the process of sexual activity, the egg and the sperm will not only represent the twenty-three chromosomes from each parent, but they will also include your emotional state and this state will be transformed to the baby and could be passed on from generation to generation, either through the physical sexual activity or through the collective karma of the society. For example, two children are born at the same time to different families. One of the children has supportive parents and is encouraged to become involved in activities. The other child is discouraged by the parents from being involved in any physical activity and will associate negativities with the activity such as 'don't swim in case you drown' or 'don't cycle in case you fall and break your leg'. This is inducing a state of fear on the child down to cellular level and it will become part of their physical makeup as a human and will also become part of their emotional tissue and will match the saying 'your issue in your issue'.

From a practical aspect and oriental point of view, the movement of your eyes represents the emotional and psychological state of your internal mind which represents your behaviour, thought and action. The physical aspect of the tongue as a muscle represents the structural aspect of your internal organs from a western and physiology perspective. The eyes are said to be the window of the soul and spirit. The state of your mind is very strongly linked to your soul, spirit, subconscious and heart. The heart in this context is not the physical aspect of the heart from physiology and western perspective such as the atrium and ventricle, instead, it is the non-physical and non-tangible aspect of the heart which is deeper down to cellular level. The movement of your eyes represents the activation of a certain part in your brain which is related to processing and functioning like when you are gathering or processing information or learning a new language. This leads to the following conclusion, our eyes from an anatomy and physiology perspective are the same for every human, but each one of us has a different way of learning which suits the movement of our eyes which is linked to our subconscious level, there are various learning styles.

Some people can learn by hearing, these are called auditory learners, they might hear something once and can repeat it all. This means the activation of their auditory cell and nerve through their brain is much stronger and influential on their memory, concentration and focus.

Some people learn by visualisation which is by looking. They might look at something once and they can remember it. This is called a photographic memory. From an oriental perspective, the reason for this is because the liver opens into the eyes and its paired organ the gallbladder is responsible for giving us our sense of direction. This is the non-physical sense of direction related to making the right decision at the right time without hesitation and regret. The physical sense of direction is when you take a person to a house and they see the location and the road is one and ten years later they can take you to the same place without any map or physical signs. This is also related to the optic nerve and to the certain cell which is responsible for the usual memory.

The third type of learning is through the sense of touch. These are called kinesthetic learners. These people prefer to write to learn and they will also prefer practicality because they will use their sense of touch. All of the senses – sight, hearing, smell, touch, taste – are all strongly linked and connected. Each sense can compensate for the other. For example, if a person is blind, regardless of whether they were born blind or as a result of an accident, the power of their sight will be transferred to their sense of hearing. Also if a person is hard of hearing or mute the power of the hearing and speech will be transferred to the other senses.

From an oriental perspective, to explain the process of taking an x-ray of the mind, if we bring two people together and give them pen and paper and ask them to sit and look at the same object such as the wall, one of them might say the wall is very nice and the colour is nice and the other person might say the wall is not nice. You ask yourself why two people looking at the same object and each of them describes it differently or has a different opinion or point of view on the object. This leads to the following conclusion, we do not see with our physical eyes and we do not hear with our physical ears. This means most of our actions, behaviour and thoughts are linked to our internal state and to the state of our mind which is linked to our eyes, tongue and heart and pericardium sac. The pericardium sac surrounds our heart and stores all of our emotions and circulates them through the blood to all of our body parts and organs.

The brain and the mind work through the three-following process:

a) Generalisation - A generalisation is when a person complains that the weather is windy or bad or raining. The same person will also complain when the weather gets hot. This means the weather is not bad because it is wet, windy or hot, it means the person has a pre-notion in their mind and generalised ideas about everything. This person does not keep their mind open and has a narrow-minded and tunnel vision view on things. This applies to every aspect of their life and not only the weather.

b) Deletion - If we ask ourselves how many sad occasions we have had in our lives or how many times people have made us angry in our lives, the answer is probably many times. If our mind and brain do not delete or help us to forget without memorising and analysing these times none of us will be able to function at all. We will be emotionally paralysed which is much harder and more destroying than the physical paralysis because even though you might be disabled in a wheelchair you might still be a genius and a creative person.

c) Distortion - Distortion is one of the most important processes in our brain and in our mind, if we think we see with our visible eye and hear with our visible ears then we are wrong. This is because these senses are inert and are influenced by the state and frequency of our mind and metabolic rate of our mind. This is not the metabolic rate related to calories and losing weight. These are the non-physical calories. For example, two people see a car accident in front of their physical eyes and each of them describes the accident differently, we ask ourselves from an oriental perspective why their visible eyes see the same accident and describe it differently? The eyes and hearing as a sense will be influenced by the state of the mind of these two people at the time the accident took place. Both people are physically standing and watching however their minds are completely and totally in different places. Another example is when a person sits and reads a newspaper, but their mind is 'somewhere else' or when a person looks at you and talks to you but their mind is 'somewhere else'. This means the concentration and focus are diverted from their physical eyes and ears is gone and connected deeper down on a cellular level to the state of their mind.

From an oriental perspective we have three minds:

Positive Mind

The positive mind is the type of mind where ideas and theories are not based on reality or fact. This mind is based on delusional scenarios that are created by the person. This will depend on what stage of your life you are at. The title of positive mind seems a good title however from an oriental perspective the positive mind leads a person to catastrophic disaster and will lead them astray from what they want to achieve regardless of what the achievement is related to. For example, when we fall in love our positive mind will be in charge of our emotion and behavioural state and the part in our brain which is responsible for making the right choices and choosing the right person. This part of the brain is linked to our sixth sense from an oriental perspective and gives us our sense of intuition and perception. When we fall in love this part of the brain in the frontal lobe will be blindfolded like a curtain coming down to block out eyes. This is what makes us hear and see what we want to hear and see when we fall in love. For example, a woman might say that the man she has fallen in love with is the best man she has ever met. This judgment is not made on logic or based on reality, but it is influenced by the state of being blindfolded and being lost inside yourself. This is why after a while when the curtain is lifted and the eyes are no longer blindfolded and the judgment part in the front lobe of the head is opened again these two people will start to see the reality of the situation and the person they started the relationship with. They then realise this is not the right person for them. This type of mind, the positive mind, does not have the balance to see the true picture and so the person ends up making the wrong decisions or choices. The picture should be based on yin and yang and should be balanced. The mind is not based on reality, it is based on delusional thoughts, this will cause the person to choose the scenario which fits their emotional and psychological criteria. Generally speaking, this type of mind is prevalent in adolescents and they will usually grow out of this state of mind however sometimes it stays with them into the next stage of their lives. People with a positive mind are the type of people who take risks. They make rash decisions without thinking about the consequences of their actions and behaviour. Generally speaking, people with a positive mind might be naïve and gullible because they see only the positive side and because they trust people without taking the time to build a realistic judgement. However, at the end of the day, we are only human and none of us are perfect or infallible.

Negative Mind

This is the mind the sees only the negative side of people and situations. It can be compared to the saying 'the glass is always half empty'. From an oriental perspective, however, the glass is half empty but the other half is filled with air and there is no such thing as half empty which means the glass is always full. Generally speaking, all of us including me have a tendency towards the negative mind more than the positive mind. This is not being pessimistic. For example, if you give someone a white t-shirt and there is a very tiny black dot on the shirt and you ask the person what do they see, the first thing the person will tell you is 'hey, see the black dot'. Why did the person not see the two pictures or why did they not say they see a nice white shirt, but they prefer the black dot not be there? At the time the person looked at the shirt it represented their negative internal state of mind which is the person having a narrow mindedness and tunnel vision perspective, so they only see what they want to see.

Neutral Mind

The neutral mind is the type of mind which creates the balance between the yin and the yang at any stage and time. This is the mind which can see the true picture of a person or a situation. For example, a woman comes into the clinic complaining about her husband after arguing with him. When I ask her how long they are together she tells me they are together twenty years. I say to her 'it's impossible during these twenty years together you have not had happy times'. If she told me they have not had any happy times together then she is with the wrong person from the start. What makes them stay together for twenty years? In this case, the situation and the argument along with the state of anger, frustration and general emotional state will influence the state of the woman's mind. It will activate and provoke the negative mind which is the mind that sees only the negative picture. Why doesn't the woman say that yes, her husband is mean, but he is also kind? In this way, she would have seen the two sides. This applies to every situation whether it is work or study etc.

Generally speaking, the neutral mind will make judgements, but this judgement is not against the human. Instead, it is against human behaviour. For example, John is a liar and Sarah is a thief, the negative mind will say that John is a liar and Sarah is a thief because the negative mind is not willing to see the good side of them. Yes, Sarah might be a thief, but she is still a kind person and John might be a liar, but he is still a generous person. We want to change their behaviour, but we do not want to change their character because you will never be able to change a person's character if they do not want to change themselves. The problem with people who are influenced by their negative mind is that they can blame and criticise others very easily but they are not willing to help these people. The neutral mind can see situations in a well-balanced scale. If you talk about a happy situation the language you use along with the tone of your voice will match your physical and emotional feeling. If the situation requires you to be on hundred per cent happy you will be one hundred per cent happy and if the situation requires you to be one hundred per cent sad you will be one hundred per cent sad. We call it an emotional electrocardiogram. If you go for a heart check-up, you might go through the process of having an electrocardiogram done. This will examine the heart physically from an anatomy and physiology perspective including the heartbeat and rhythm. However, from an oriental perspective the heart captures the mind and the pericardium, the muscular sac surrounding the heart, holds all our emotions. As the heart circulates the blood and the blood captures the mind it will capture the state of your three minds, the positive, the negative and neutral. The frequency and rhythm of the heartbeat from an emotional aspect will depend on which mind you are at which will influence your heart rate and beat. This can be explained using the negative mind and the lungs as an example. The lungs are related to sadness and grief and the tissue they control is the skin. If a person is sad for a long period this will lead to depression. This state of depression will vary from person to person for example; some people will depression will often have very low blood pressure however others with depression often have very high blood pressure. Sometimes the medication that these people take play a major role in the relapse and remission of their condition in general and the relapse and remission of the heart as an organ from an oriental perspective. When the blood pressure changes from very low to very high it influences the physical strength and capacity of the person and also the energy of the whole body. This is why some people with depression will sleep for 24 hours a day, not leave the house or do any physical activity, they don't have any social or emotional interaction and if they do it will be influenced and affected by their negative mind. On the other hand, there are people with depression who are not able to sleep at all. They could be hyperactive and their mind will always be wandering and racing and even when they go to bed their physical body is resting their mind will be racing and jumping from idea to idea. From an oriental perspective the blood captures the mind, the mind is controlled by the heart and the mind is related to our subconscious. We cannot sleep without going deep down to the cellular level and the subconscious level.

From an oriental perspective, there are two types of insomnia. The first type is when the person can't fall asleep to start with; this is caused by blood deficiency and can sometimes occur in people with anaemia or in people whose bodies are lacking nutrients in general. The second type is when the person can fall asleep but they wake up in the middle of the night and cannot go back to sleep and while they are awake their mind is creating scenarios, thoughts and ideas and eventually, these will turn to emotional feelings and over a long period this will turn to physical feelings such as fear which will affect your kidneys and you might have butterfly feelings which will affect your stomach.

The positive mind is related to joy, happiness and excitement which is linked and hugely connected to the heart. This can be proved because from an oriental perspective we say that the heart rhythm and beat is influenced by your emotional state. From an oriental perspective, we call it an emotional electrocardiogram. Ask yourself this question, when you are happy or excited, what happens to your heart? The heart beats faster because the emotional state of happiness, excitement or joy affects the rhythm of the heart and this is connected to your positive of mind.

The Upper Jiao is the area in the body where the respiratory system is located along with the lungs as an organ and the heart as an organ. The lungs are related to sadness and grief and the heart is related to joy, excitement and happiness. The imbalance between these two energies, the lung energy and the heart energy as organs and the emotional energy related to sadness and happiness, will be influenced by our state of mind at any time and in any situation. For example, you might have heard of people who hear happy news and they 'drop dead' with a heart attack, similarly, you might have heard of people who 'drop dead' when they hear bad news. From an oriental perspective, this represents the imbalance between the yin and yang from a structural, functional, emotional, psychological and sexual aspect. The main function of the neutral mind is to create the perfect imbalance for feelings to come without causing any disaster so that the feelings do not manifest suddenly and abruptly leading to potential sudden death, this applies to every situation.

It is the function of the neutral mind to create a balance, regardless of what condition we have. It is our job as oriental practitioners to go back to the root cause of the client's problems to create the perfect balance from every aspect. This is what we mean when we say life is built on the five elements and the yin and the yang.

The Heart from a Five Element Perspective

Season – Summer

The heart represents summer as a season. The reason for this is because the heart represents the stage of youth in life. The youth and adolescent stage of life is active and full of movement. All of these physical activities produce heat which explains why the heart represents summer as a season. The heart is hugely connected to our emotional state and feelings and the growth stage of our life from a western perspective is connected to the production of our hormones and the stage of 'growing up'. This explains why during this stage we are not influenced or controlled by our brain or logic, especially from s female aspect. For a female, this is the time when her period and ovulation will start. Both of these processes will have a huge impact on her feelings, thinking and thought. When girls are having pre-menstrual symptoms, these symptoms are triggered and influenced by Liver Qi. The liver energy comes like waves from the sea and this is what makes the girl's mood fluctuate between yin and yang. This explains why when the girl is having pre-menstrual symptoms, she will laugh at something and ten minutes later she will cry at the same thing. There are two reasons for this, firstly because the liver energy is like a wave when the energy is receding the girls will mot be affected and influenced by things and will not react to it. Secondly, it depends on where the girl is at emotionally and at what stage of mind, they are in. If they are in a neutral mind, they won't react but if they are in a negative mind when something is said to them, they will have a negative response and reaction to it. If they are in a positive mind, they will have a positive reaction and response however from an oriental perspective this reaction, from a positive mind, will lead to catastrophic disaster because it allows the person to be easily influenced and led by others. The person's intentions are good but the outcome and consequences which come after the intention will be bad.

As I mentioned earlier the neutral mind will be in control of your body, thoughts, actions and behaviour at any stage and time throughout your life but especially at the time of menstruation and ovulation. This is because the neutral mind is related to the cosmos which is the collected karma to the entire universe. Everything in the universe is one and this is the oneness of everything and everything in the universe is connected and linked to the moon and sun. Changes in the moon can affect all, regardless of gender. The moon is yin and represents night and the sun is yang and represents the day. Movement and fluctuation in changing from night to day and from day to night will affect everything in the universe including our health and emotional state. The movement of the moon and the sun will determine the minutes, days, weeks, months and seasons in our life. Seconds will turn into minutes, minutes to hours, twelve hours together represent half the day and at this stage, the day starts to turn from yin to yang. Nothing is in a static state. Daytime turns into night and night-time turns into day, the cold turns into heat and heat turns into cold, two sets of twelve hours from the day consisting of twenty-four hours, a group of days form the month, a group of months form the season. As we said the heart represents the summer season. This seasonal change will affect all the processes in our body including our emotional state and our wellbeing and bodily functions particularly the endocrine system which is related to our hormones which control our state of mind and plays a major role in our healing and recovery. This explains why people will go on holidays to a hot country and they will feel a lot better without any treatment whether from an oriental perspective or a western perspective. The best example is people who have asthma or arthritis, the damp cold and windy weather may make the condition worse if they have osteoarthritis which is opposite to rheumatoid arthritis. The reason for this is because osteoarthritis is a cold condition related to degeneration of the joint and anything connected and linked to the joint such as the ligament, cartilage, tendon, tissue and synovial fluid which is the slimy lubricant fluid that fills the joint and prevents frictions between bones. Osteoarthritis is regarded as a cold condition from an oriental perspective because it is caused by stagnation of qi, lymph, fluid, yin and yang. The synovial fluid is the yin and the movement of the fluid is yang. This in return will lead to stagnation of blood which from a western perspective represents your circulation and particularly the circulation in the extremities. This will be explained further when I talk about the functions of the spleen, one of which is to push the qi upward which represents the venous return of the blood to the heart, this means the return of the de-oxygenated blood from the lower limbs to the heart and from the heart to the lungs to be oxygenated again and the cycle goes on. The reason why people with osteoarthritis feel better when they go to a hot country is that the heat from the sun helps their joints and circulation and will also help their hormones which will help their emotional state. Also, vitamin D from the sun will help the mind and brain and speed up the healing and recovery process from their condition.

The day which consists of twenty-four hours will be linked to the twelve channels that are in our body. As I mentioned earlier the energy passes every two hours from yin and yang channels. For example, the channel goes from lungs to large intestine after two hours. From an oriental perspective, we call this the biological transformation and transportation of the yin and the yan and it is also known as the biological clock of human physical pain. For example, you could have a toothache at any time of the day or night but in the night the toothache always gets worse, because the night represents the state of rest and it needs the hormones which are responsible for the state of rest and because you ate your three meals during the day your gastric juices have been used in the digestion of the food. The gastric juices are the yin aspect of your stomach from an oriental perspective and they are equivalent to the adrenaline and endorphin as a hormone which influences your state of calmness and the state of wellbeing which is opposite to the state of being in pain.

A group of four seasons come together to form a year. The year as three hundred and sixty-five days. These days will be influenced and affected by the movement of the sun and the moon. The mood and the sun influence our weather and the tides of the ocean. This is what causes the eclipse and also the leap year where there is an extra day every four years. These changes will have an impact on our health and wellbeing in addition to our lifestyle affecting our health and wellbeing.

Groups of years come together to form different stages of our life. The first seven years are childhood years. Years eight to fourteen are the adolescent years, another stage of life. Years fifteen to twenty-one you are becoming an adult and you have all your future ahead of you. The fourth stage is the years from twenty-two to twenty-eight and during this stage, you are fully grown, and you might want to start to a family. The next stage is from twenty-nine to thirty-five, in this stage, your mind and your brain are more in control of your physical body and are more in control of your desires.

From a female aspect the younger the woman is when she has the children the more likely it is that she will have a healthy pregnancy, normal labour and healthy baby. The longer the woman waits to have children it will decrease the possibility of becoming pregnant. The sixth stage is from the years thirty-six to forty-two, now you have your own family. The seventh stage is from the age forty-three to forty-nine, during this stage your hair will start to grey, and your memory will start to decline especially your short-term memory. The next stage is from fifty-seven to sixty-three, this is the retirement age and stage of rest. Elderly people do activities which are not always related to physical movement such as playing cards. The next stage of life is from sixty-four to seventy. During this stage, our perception on life starts to change completely. We start to think about what life is all about similar to a pregnant woman when she knows she is getting closer to her 40th week of pregnancy she knows the inevitably she is getting closer to her labour and delivery of a new-born baby. The same process takes place in our mind when we are at this stage if life. We are all on the same journey in this life regardless of our beliefs. As we began our life in the womb in a dark place we will go to the grave to a dark place. However, because death is not the conclusion this means this only the physical death, when the body physically ceases to function, we will be reborn again but this time in a different form of life.

The next life is completely different from this life. Our bodies are not designed to live forever. Our physical body and our physical senses have limitations which are related to size and measurement and also to time. The next life does not have physical limitations related to shape, size, measurement or time.

From an oriental perspective, you have your sense of hearing and you have your sense of sight; both of these senses have a physical limitation designed for this life. For example, if you take somebody to a quiet and spacious place such as the desert and you play loud music and you ask them to start walking away from the music you will find that after they walk beyond a certain distance they will still be able to hear the music but not as clearly as before when they walk further again they will not be able to hear the music at all. In this case, the music is still playing at the same volume and the person still has the same capacity of hearing, but the hearing has a physical limitation related to the distance. The same principle applies to the sense of sight. If you ask a person to walk away from you in a straight line you will be able to see them to a certain distance, then they will become smaller and eventually you will be no longer able to see them, this is the physical limitation of our sight. These limitations can also be applied to our strength and speed however these limitations do not exist in the next life because the next life is related to our soul and spirit, as I mentioned earlier our soul and our spirit are weightless, timeless, they are infinite.

Taste – Bitter

The heart as an organ controls the bitter taste. Earlier I spoke about two different types of people, the liver person and the heart person. The heart person is a bitter person and the feelings and behaviours of bitterness will affect the heart person's sense of taste. If we exclude any structural or physical condition the heart person will have a bitter taste in their mouth. The reason for this from an oriental perspective is because as I said earlier every aspect of the world is built on the yin and yang, this applies to all of our physical feelings, senses and emotions. If we look at it as a sense of taste the spleen controls the sweet taste and the spleen from an oriental perspective represents the heart and the hearts circulation from a western perspective because the spleen has to carry and hold the energy for twenty-four hours. The opposite taste to the sweet taste is the bitter taste. Therefore, because the heart controls the circulation and the heart controls the bitter taste the heart person will have a bitter taste which is opposite to the spleen.

Direction – South

The south represents the heat and represents summertime. The summertime is the time when everything becomes ripe. the heart represents the growing up of the body and therefore represents the youth. When we are in the youth stage of our lives we think with our heart and with our emotional feelings and sexual desires more than we think with our logic and common sense by a general standard.

Sound – Loud

As a sound, the heart represents a loud sound. When we are youths we talk very loud. The loud sound is related to heat. This explains why people from such hot countries talk very loudly and they also use their arms a lot to express themselves such as the people from the Middle East who will be opposite to people from Norway or another cold country who will talk very low and in a calm manner. To apply it from a western perspective and a medical condition we will consider hyperthyroidism and hypothyroidism. Hyperthyroidism is an overactive thyroid. The hyper represents the activity, the body is producing lots of thyroxine. The function of the thyroxine is to regulate the metabolic rate and the person will eat a lot and their heart rate will be very fast. The person will also be very thin no matter how much they eat. All of these symptoms are a sign of hyperactivity from a western perspective and a yang excess from an oriental perspective which means excess heat. This excess heat in return will demolish the yin whose function is to cool and moisture and in return, it will create even more heat. Too much thyroxine will affect the gastric juices of the stomach which are equivalent to the yin from an oriental perspective and will demolish them. When the gastric juices are demolished there will be a sense of emptiness in the body particularly in the stomach as an organ and the digestive as a system. This explains why the person with this condition will eat a lot because they are to fill this emptiness. Hypothyroid is an underactive thyroid where the body is not producing sufficient thyroxine. This person will have yang deficiency where the heat aspect of the person is decreased. This explains why people with this condition will feel very cold most of the time especially in the extremities and especially in their feet. The person might also have puffy eyes, swollen ankles and will be bloated and will put on weight even when they don't eat a lot, they will also have a pale complexion and in most cases, they will have low blood pressure. It will be very rare for these people to get headaches and even if they do get a headache the headache will be different and will not be a form of migraine, tinnitus or vertigo which are all related to excess, instead the headache will be dull and they will feel it more so in the night-time and they might describe it as feeling like a band around the forehead or squeezing the forehead. As the evening goes on their mental capacity, strength and memory will decrease a lot. As I said earlier yang is day and represents heat and activity and yin is night and represents rest, sleep and the dropping of the heart rate and body temperature which makes the person feel colder and will add to their condition as they already have the yang deficiency. The treatment that these people receive will be different from the treatment received by people with hyperthyroidism where there is too much heat. In the case of hyperthyroidism, we use a specific acupuncture point in the body to expel heat from all the body but especially from the affected meridian and organ and we also nourish the yin to cool and moisture and pull the yang down. We also ask people with excess heat to eat foods that have a cooling effect on the body's cells and tissues such as food that contain a lot of enzymes like lettuce, cucumber and beetroot. The person with hypothyroidism will receive a treatment to expel cold and heat the body. We also ask these people to use a hot water bottle on their chest, lower back and on the kidney area on the back particularly between the two kidneys on the place we call the 'gate of vitality'. This is the same area where a lumbar puncture is performed for a meningitis test or where an epidural is administered. These people are also asked to avoid cold drinks however generally speaking every one of us should avoid cold drinks or anything below room temperature as it will affect and damage our circulation and undermines the function of the spleen from an oriental perspective and the heart from a western perspective. The reason for this is because when we drink the cold drink, we are causing a sudden shock on the body and organs. The kidneys from an oriental perspective are related to shock, any kind of shock regardless of the reason for it, by drinking the cold drink it creates a shock to the body particularly the kidney and the heart.

From a western perspective, if we have a kidney failure, we will also have a heart failure and vice versa.

In one of my workshops, I was asked by someone from a medical background how this could be proved from an oriental perspective and I gave him the following example if the weather is very hot and you give one person icy cold water to drink and another person water at room temperature to drink, which one of them will feel the heat more and which one of them will sweat more? The response immediately was the person who drank the icy cold water. This is because the person who drank the icy cold water has to work harder to maintain the balance between the interior and the exterior environment to regulate the body temperature. When the weather is hot the skin pores open to allow the sweat to evaporate to regulate the temperature. When the weather is cold the pores close and the hair on the skin stand up to protect the body heat and to preserve the heat. As I mentioned earlier the kidneys are related to shock, any kind of shock, if you are lost in a cold place your body will start to shiver and tries to protect you from the shock and tries to maintain the temperature, this is an example of physical shock. An example of emotional shock is if you hear bad news the hair on your skin stands up, commonly known as 'goosebumps' and the body tries to protect itself to cope with the emotional shock and the emotional feelings which all of your body's systems and organs are bombarded with suddenly and abruptly. Because the kidney is related to shock if the body is not able to cope it will lead to kidney and in return it will lead to heart failure. Both the kidney and the skin have the function of regulating body fluid. The kidney excretes fluid through the bladder as a form of urine and the skin excretes the fluid through the process of expelling and evaporating which takes place when you sweat. Finally, people who have hypothyroidism have a very low and weak voice. This is because there is a weakness in their circulation and their lungs. One of the functions of the lung is to produce qi and the voice and the location of the vocal cord in the neck is in the same area as the thyroid gland. People with hyperthyroidism are the opposite with loud voices and they are not afraid to express themselves and they will say what they feel. Sometimes people with hypothyroidism might also have depression and this is related to the balance between the yin and yang from an oriental perspective. Our job as a practitioner is to bring balance to these people and any other medical condition whether it is from an emotional, physical, sexual or mental aspect.

Colour – Red

The colour red represents the heart and the heart represents the red colour. There are two reasons for this from an oriental perspective. Firstly, the heart circulates blood around all of the body and as you know the colour of blood is red. Secondly, the heart represents the south as a direction from a five-element point of view and the south represents the sun which represents the heat which is represented by the colour red. Heat is created by activity and activity is created by heat. For example, when you run the colour of your face, especially your cheeks, will be red. From an oriental perspective, the heart is a yin organ and has a yang job to do. The more activity there is the more there will be which means more circulation. The more circulation there is the redder your complexion will be. If you don't move there is no activity and there will stagnation so you will pale. As I mentioned above the heart represents the youth stage and it also represents the south.

Opposite to this is the kidney which represents the north, cold and old age. The older we become the less active we are and the colder we will be. This explains why some elderly people look paler than usual and in the youth sage people look red and rosy, especially in the face after activity.

CHAPTER 6

PATTERNS OF THE HEART

Heart Qi Deficiency

This represents the functional aspect of the heart from an anatomy and physiology perspective. As we said earlier qi pushes blood and blood nourishes qi. If heart qi is deficient, especially for long periods, this leads to the weakness of the heart from a functional and structural aspect.

Signs and symptoms:

➢ Palpitations or irregular heartbeat. This is because qi is so deficient or weak and is not able to keep up the rhythm and the beat of the heart at regular intervals.

➢ Shortness of breath which becomes worse with physical exertion or exercise. This is because the person is not able to get enough oxygen with each breath. The breathing becomes shallow in this case and there might be more carbon dioxide invading the body than oxygen.

➢ The pulse will be very weak and slow in severe cases is very hard to find.

➢ The heart circulates blood around all of the body and the heart opens into the tongue, when there is not enough blood the tongue will look pale.

Heart Yang Deficiency

Heart Qi deficiency for a long period leads to heart yang deficiency.

The function of yin is to cool and moisture. The function of yang is to push up, circulate, and warm which represents the circulation from a western perspective. The saying 'warm hands cold hands' relates to circulation when there is not enough heart yang.

Signs and symptoms:

➤ The person will have a cold in their body but especially in their hands and feet.

➤ The lips will be blue and dark in colour due to stagnation.

➤ Excess sweating.

This condition over a long period can lead to excess sweating especially during the daytime this is because the night is yin and the day is yang. One of the hearts functions from an oriental perspective is to control sweating and there will not be enough yang to push the fluid up to keep it in the body and also there will be a weakness in the defensive qi which means weakness in the immune system which in return is not able to close the skin pores meaning the person will sweat profoundly. The more the person sweats the more the body will lose its vital substances which in return will affect the person's mind because one of the functions of the heart is to capture the mind and if the mind is not captured the person will be confused and distracted and will not be in a stable mental state.

Aetiology of Heart Qi and Heart Yang Deficiency

Many causative factors contribute to heart qi deficiency and heart yang deficiency

- ➢ Chronic illness for a long period
- ➢ Taking drugs for a long period
- ➢ Mental and psychological strains and emotional issues for a long period leading to unhappiness. This is because the heart controls happiness, joy, and excitement as emotions and in return, the heart will pay the price for your emotional feelings and the state of your mind but especially the qi and yang will be affected.

Heart Yin Deficiency

As we the function of the yin is to cool and moisture. One of the heart's functions is to circulate the blood around all of the body's systems and organs down to the cellular level. The blood is a form of fluid and a form of yin and vice versa. Hence the function of the blood is to cool and moisture. Blood is a part of yin and yin is a part of blood. If there is heart yin deficiency for a long period this will lead to heart blood deficiency and this is why both heart yin deficiency and heart blood deficiency share almost the same signs and symptoms.

Signs and symptoms:

- ➢ Palpitations and irregular heartbeat.

  This can occur during the day but will get worse at night because the day is yang and night is yin and there will not be enough heart yin particularly in the night-time.

➢ Unable to maintain a peaceful nights sleep

One of the functions of the heart is to capture the mind. The mind is the non-physical aspect of the brain which is responsible for taking the person to the subconscious stage. This is the stage that is required for the sleeping process and if you are unable to fall asleep in the first place it means you have blood deficiency especially heart blood deficiency. This explains why some people with anaemia are unable to sleep at all because there is not enough blood to capture their mind and to stop it from wandering around and creating delusional scenarios that are not based on reality. The reason for this from a western perspective is that there is not enough iron or oxygen reaching the brain and subsequently this leads to a chemical imbalance in the brain. This chemical imbalance leads to a hormonal imbalance which leads to insomnia. The function of our body's hormones is to control our body's functions from a physical aspect and to control our emotional state and the state of our mind which is very important for the sleeping process especially by producing the hormones from the gland which represents our third eye chakra to help us with our sleeping process. If you can fall asleep easily but you are not able to maintain your sleep this means you have yin deficiency, especially heart yin deficiency because there will not be enough yin to maintain the sleep process and even when you sleep, a short period of your sleep will be disturbed by visual or frightening dreams because there will not be enough heart yin to capture the mind for you while you are asleep. From an oriental perspective, your mind needs to be captured whether you are awake or asleep.

- Mental restlessness and mental confusion

  Every emotion is linked to the heart. If your mind is not captured you will have mental restlessness and you will find it difficult to find a comfortable position at night in bed and you will be twisting and turning and doing a lot of twisting, turning, jerking, and moving while you are asleep.

- Heat in the blood

  Not enough heart yin means there is not enough coolness in the blood and the blood will be overheated. The heart will pump this overheated blood around of the body but especially the face and sometimes the sole of the feet and the palms of the hands which explains why the person may become more irritable at night-time and sometimes they will have a low-grade fever with a red face and they might sweat from the armpit and the soles of the feet and the palms of the hands will be clammy.

  Women going through the menopause stage might have some of these symptoms in addition to a bitter taste in their mouth. The reason for this is because estrogen is yin and has the function to cool and moisture and progesterone is yang and has the function to warm and push. If the woman does not have enough estrogen to cool and moisture, they will have the symptoms mentioned above.

- The tongue will be red which is a sign of heat and is caused by yin deficiency.

- The pulse will be fast but empty because there will not be enough yin to fill the vessels during the circulations process which is controlled by the heart.

Heart Blood Stagnation

If heart qi and heart yang deficiency exist the qi will no longer be able to push the blood and the heart blood will become stagnant.

Signs and symptoms:

> Palpitations - The stagnation leads to palpitations because the heart continues to work hard to keep the blood moving.

> Piercing or bracing pain especially on the left side of the chest where the heart is located. If the stagnation has existed for a long period the pain can become so severe that it starts to travel to the back and the shoulder, especially the left shoulder. The reason for this is the heart is a yin organ and its paired yang organ is the small intestine, there is a point on the small intestine channel called small intestine 19, and it lies under the shoulder blade where the scapula is located, the function of this point is to manufacture blood and that explains why the heart affects the shoulder and the shoulder affects the heart. This indicates the importance of good posture. If you slouch a lot will cause the qi to stagnate, especially the heart qi and the lung qi. Because qi pushes blood and blood nourishes qi this function will become impaired which results in the symptoms being a lot worse.

> Blue or dark lips and nails

> When qi and blood are stagnant and not moving to the extremities the nails will look blue or dark.

> The tongue will be blue and purple and sometimes there may also be raised spots.

> The pulse might miss a beat because the heart qi is stagnant.

➤ Aetiology of Heart Blood Stagnation

➤ Mental strain over a long period causes heart qi to become stagnant and heart qi will not move heart blood and the blood will become stagnant. Over a long period this will lead to anxiety and in severe cases can lead to depression.

➤ Using medication for a long period will weaken the heart qi so the heart is no longer able to circulate the blood around the body efficiently and the blood will become stagnant.

➤ Injuries such as a kick or being hit by a fist or a ball will also cause the qi and blood to become stagnant. Another example is when you twist your ankle and the qi and blood become stagnant on the affected area. This will result in a bruise and inflammation the swollen effect of the joint. Generally speaking, any stagnation of the blood is caused by weakness of the yang qi, especially the heart yang qi. That is why the person will have chest pains especially on the left side and sometimes the pain will travel down the left arm to the ring finger and little finger in the hand where the heart channel ends.

Heart Fire Blazing

Generally speaking, this condition is caused by mental, psychological, and emotional problems for a long period. The reason for this is because the mental, psychological and emotional strain and being in a state of not being happy and being depressed for a long period will damage the heart yin and at the same time will damage all of the yin in our body in general. As we now know, the function of the yin is to cool and moisture. If there is not enough yin to cool and moisture this will allow the heat to build up in the body and this heat goes down to blood level which will cause further damage to the heart yin and the heart blood. The heart will pump this heat and fire around the body.

Signs and symptoms:

➢ Swollen mouth and tongue. The heart opens into the tongue.

➢ Mouth ulcers

➢ Bleeding from the mouth and lips

➢ Bitter taste in the mouth. The heart controls the bitter taste

➢ Insomnia. The heart is unable to capture the mind resulting in insomnia

➢ The feeling of heat similar to having a temperature, especially in the face. The person will look redder than usual.

➢ Dark yellow and strong-smelling urine - This is because the heart goes down to the kidney and the kidney also leads to the heart and so the two are connected which is why from a western perspective if you have kidney failure you will have heart failure and vice versa.

➢ The tongue will be red

➢ Pulse will be very fast and rapid - This is because the heart is causing hyperactivity in all of the body systems and organs. This hyperactivity will especially affect the heart's function hence the pulse will be very fast.

Phlegm and Fire Misting the Mind

This is one of the most serious conditions related to the heart from an oriental medicine perspective because the signs and symptoms that the person produces and shows are all an indication of a mental and psychological condition.

Signs and symptoms:

> The person will have mental depression and will be in a state of dullness and confusion. This is caused by the stagnation of the body's qi in general but especially the heart qi. If heart qi is stagnant it will not be able to push the blood, yin, and fluids. This stagnation of the blood, yin, and fluids will cause the phlegm to build up. This is not the form of phlegm that is related to the lungs that you could cough up when you have a cold or flu, this phlegm is like a form of fog or steam which will mist the mind and cause mental confusion and lack of clarity of the mind.

> The person's actions and behavior can be uncontrollable because the phlegm is misting the mind. For example, laughing suddenly and abruptly for no particular reason at inappropriate times or crying and screaming and being in an upset state at inappropriate times.

> Slurred or incoherent speech can occur in severe cases - This is because the heart opens into the tongue and controls speech.

> Fainting and coma can occur in extremely severe cases and may lead to death. The reason for this is because if the phlegm heat and phlegm fire sink into the pericardium, the muscular sac surrounding the heart, it causes a massive amount of heat which turns into a fever. This fever causes the person to be in a state of delirium which destroys the

mind completely and causes a coma that the person will not come out of. This could eventually lead to death.

CHAPTER 7

THE FUNCTION OF THE SPLEEN

From an oriental perspective the spleen has six functions:
1) Transformation and transportation
2) Makes blood
3) Holds qi in place
4) Controls the 65 muscles in especially the extremities
5) Opens into the lips
6) Controls the memory

Before going through the functions in detail I want to clarify something, when we say the spleen, we do not mean the structural aspect of the spleen, instead, we mean the function and emotional aspect of the spleen as an organ from an oriental perspective.

The spleen is yin organ and it has a yang job to do. Its paired organ is the stomach. The spleen from an oriental perspective represents the heart from a western perspective. The function of the heart is to constantly pump blood around the blood. One of the functions of the spleen is to constantly push the qi upward from the toes to the head. This represents the venous return of the de-oxygenated blood to the heart and the lungs where it is re-oxygenated again through the process of breathing and the interaction between the lungs, the heart, the liver, and the stomach.

1) Transformation and Transportation

Transportation

The word transportation means to move from place to place. This transportation represents the physical aspect of the human body like you are travelling from town to town. From an oriental perspective, the word transportation has a broader meaning. The spleen transports the energy, fluid, lymph, and blood around all of the body's systems and organs down to the tissue and cellular level.

From a western perspective, this represents the movement and transportation of the interstitial fluid between tissues, cells, and organs. As I mentioned earlier the world is built on the five elements and the yin and the yang from every perspective and this can be applied to this process of transportation. From an oriental perspective the process of transportation represents the metabolic rate and the activity of the tissue down to a cellular level where every cell has to do the following:

A) Take oxygen

B) Take fluid

C) Take nutrients

D) Expel the toxin and the waste

E) Die and leave the body to be replaced by new cells

The process of taking nutrients, fluid, and oxygen is a continuous process of transportation, carrying everything around the body and down to a cellular level to keep every organ and tissue alive.

When there is no transportation there is no transformation of energy or fluid and this will lead to the death of the organ, tissue, and cell. This is from an anatomy and physiology perspective but from an oriental perspective, the reason I say transportation has a broader meaning is that the spleen controls short-term memory and it also controls focus, concentration, intellect and it controls the state of mind which represents the present moment.

Transformation

From an oriental perspective, this represents the western aspect of digestion by taking the nutrients from the food that we eat and the fluid that we drink and turning it into energy which will be stored in the liver as a form of glycogen and will be released as a form of glucose when it is required for physical activity where it will be supplied to the working muscles and organs. As we said the spleen is yin and the stomach is yang. The nutrients go to your body through the process of eating. The first organ to deal with this process after chewing the food in the mouth is the stomach. The stomach is a yang organ because it is hollow and it works when it is required, it has a yin job to do which is to produce the gastric juices and gastric enzymes to aid the digestion process. The stomach carries out this process through the process of muscular contraction, called peristalsis in western medicine, also known as 'rotting and ripening', along with a continuous movement of the stomach by contracting and relaxing. The process can be compared to being similar to a blending process when a blender is used to make a smoothie. This process is helped and determined by the function of the spleen as an organ from an oriental perspective the stronger your digestion will be in general and you will not have burping, belching, heartburn, or indigestion after eating your food. This is with the help of the liver qi, the liver is a yin organ, and the movement of the gallbladder qi which represents the production of bile, the gallbladder is the paired yang organ of the liver. As I mentioned earlier the function of the bile is to burn the fat to prevent indigestion. This explains why people who have had their gallbladder removed will experience the indigestion symptoms mentioned above. Generally speaking, the stomach prefers a wet environment and the spleen prefers a dry environment. One of the stomachs' functions is to produce the gastric juices which represent the yin aspect from an oriental perspective. As we now know the function of the yin is to cool and moisture. The normal flow of stomach qi is the descending downward of the fluid and the food towards the small intestine. The stomach is a yang organ with a yin job to do and as a direction, it is a yin direction bringing the food downward. The stomach is the center of the body and both the stomach and spleen are in the middle Jiao portion of the body. From an oriental perspective, the viscera in the body is divided into three sections, the upper Jiao which represents the heart and lungs, the middle Jiao which represents the stomach and spleen, and the lower Jiao which represents the reproductive system. From a five-element point of view, the stomach and the spleen represent the earth and the earth is in the middle between the moon and sun. Generally speaking, most of our health problems are related to our digestive system and the stomach. This coincides with the saying 'you are what you eat'. We can add another theory from an oriental perspective which is 'you are what you think'. The stomach is related to anxiety and worry. If you are in an anxious and worried state you will lose your appetite or it will decrease. This will then go further down to your senses particularly the sense of taste and as we now know the spleen controls the sense of taste. The transformation and transportation of food will be affected by your emotional state and the way you are feeling because the spleen will transport this state to all of your body's systems and organs down to the cellular level. The spleen channel starts on the medial side of the big toe and if you have gout you will have it in the big toe where the spleen channel begins. This blocked and obstruction in the spleen channel will have been there for a long period because you will not get gout in your feet overnight. To define gout, it is a form of calcification and build-up of the protein, sugar, and acid in all of the body but especially in your extremities and particularly in the big toe. The question is what is the root cause of this build-up?

The answer is that it is due to a variety of reasons including the consumption of a lot of red meat, too much oily greasy foods, too much carbohydrate, and sugar or drinking a lot of cold drinks because as I mentioned earlier any food or drink under room temperature will undermine the function of the spleen from an oriental perspective and will shock the kidneys and the heart from a western perspective. In addition to this drinking, a lot of alcohol and smoking will have a detrimental effect on the body in general, but especially on the digestive system. The eating habit will affect the stomach, alcohol will affect the liver and smoking will affect the lungs, and because all of our organs are interdependent when one organ malfunctions it will affect every other organ. Generally speaking, when a yin organ is affected its paired yang organ will pay the price first and vice versa. For example, the lung is a yin organ and its paired yang organ is the large intestine, the function of the lungs is to breathe which is activity and movement and therefore yang. The lungs also contain pleura, which is a form of fluid and represents the yin aspect, and this fluid fills the pleura cavity and prevents friction between the lungs and its surrounding environment and structure. If the person smokes this will demolish the fluid in the lungs and the cooling and moisture aspect of the lungs is either decreased or gone completely, this is called lung yin deficiency from an oriental perspective, in return, this will affect the large intestine, the paired organ to the lungs.

One of the functions of the lungs is to descend, which represents the diffusion to all of the body and particularly the skin aspect from a western perspective. It is common to see people with asthma who also have constipation. The use of drugs and inhalers over a long period will further damage and demolish the yin which in return will demolish all of the fluid in the body but particularly the skin and bowel. A healthy bowel should always be moist and wet to allow the movement of waste through it with the help of the lung function of descending and dispersing which represents the relaxation and contraction of the digestion and excretion which is the peristalsis action of the bowel from a western perspective.

How does the bowel affect the lung function from an oriental perspective? If a person consumes a lot of red meat, and a lot of hot spicy oily, and greasy food it will take a longer length of time to be digested and to be expelled out of the body which leads to further dryness and constipation. In return, the energy from the bowel will send the heat to the lungs which will be dispersed and diffused by the lungs to all of the body's systems and organs but especially the skin. This is why people with skin conditions will notice that their condition gets worse after consuming a lot of alcohol or red meat. This is because the skin is a yin organ with a yang job to do which is sweating. The skin is a yin organ with a yang job to do which is sweating. The skin contains subcutaneous glands which are yang in nature and have a yin job to do which is to produce the sebum oil whose function is to lubricate. Excessive consumption of alcohol will dry the bowel and the bowel will dry the lungs and if we want to chase the root it goes back to the stomach where the stomach yin and stomach qi has been dissolved completely. The stomach, bowel, and lungs start to diffuse heat to all of the body and particularly the skin. This explains why most conditions from an oriental perspective are related to dryness which is caused by the stomach and the large intestine. However, there can also be other causes of dryness such as excessive urination when the kidney and bladder are weakened and are not able to hold the qi and fluid for long periods. The lungs are related to sadness and grief and they control the skin, the combination of your emotional state, the combination of your emotional state, especially sadness and grief, along with your lifestyle will further worsen the condition whether it is asthma, eczema, acne, dermatitis, or constipation.

This is because the skin and the bowel share the same emotional function of letting go, the skin through the process of sweating, and the bowel through the process of expelling and excreting body waste. Some people will find out that when they go to a hot country, they will feel better, this is due to the sun, light, heat, and absorption of vitamin D through the skin because the vitamins and the heat affect your hormonal system and help your emotional state and the state of letting go.

As we said earlier any disharmony in the yin organ will affect its paired yang organ. The same thing applies to the stomach and the spleen, any disharmony or malfunction of the spleen as a yin organ will affect the function of the stomach as a yang organ. Generally speaking, if you smoke it will dry the lung yin which is equivalent to the fluid and consequently it will affect the function of the large intestine by drying the bowel which leads to constipation however with the stomach and the spleen it's the complete opposite.

Comparison of the Stomach and the Spleen

Spleen	Stomach
Yin organ with a yang job to do	Yang organ with a yin job to do
Yin organ works twenty-four hours a day	Yang organ works when required
Spleen is dense	Stomach is hollow
Spleen energy goes upwards towards the head	Stomach energy goes down
Channel begins on the big toe and ends on the ribs on the side of the chest	Channel begins below the eyelid beside the nose and ends on the second toe
Prefers dryness	Prefers wetness
Extracts the food qi	Receives the food qi
Affected by Damp and Phlegm	Affected by Damp and Phlegm
Damp and cold will undermine the spleen	Dryness and heat will undermine the stomach

Damp vs Phlegm

Damp	Phlegm
Damp is heavy, descends, affects spleen function, and accumulates in ankles and feet	Phlegm is lighter, ascends, settles on top of the hairline where the point stomach 8 is
Damp affects physical activity and strength, the state of being tired	Phlegm is lighter, ascends, settles on top of the hairline where the point stomach 8 is
	Phlegm affects the stomach and the state of your focus, concentration, memory, intellect, and alertness
Damp down is yin in nature because it descends	Phlegm is yang in nature because it descends up
Damp is caused by Spleen Qi deficiency but especially Spleen Yang Deficiency	Phlegm caused by Spleen Qi deficiency but especially Spleen Yang Deficiency

I will go through each of the comparisons above

1) Spleen is a yin organ with a yang job to do; Stomach is a yang organ with a yin job to do

The spleen from an oriental perspective represents the heart by constantly pushing energy around the body to the systems and organs. From an oriental perspective, the food qi is extracted from the food with the help of the spleen function. From a western perspective, the heart has to send blood to the stomach to start the digestion process. If you stand for long periods and you feel tired this will affect your digestion in general but especially the stomach because one of the functions of the spleen is to control the four extremities, the arms, and legs, and to control the muscular strength and standing for long periods the spleen energy is exhausted which leads to spleen qi deficiency which consequently leads to stomach qi deficiency and stomach yin deficiency. This is why when people feel tired and exhausted, they either have no appetite at all or else they do not have the energy to eat. If you eat a lot of salad, raw food, and cold food or drink icy cold drinks this will undermine the spleen and will create an environment for bloated-ness, swollen ankles, puffy legs, and puffiness under the eyes. Also, consuming a lot of hot spicy oily greasy food will damage the stomach by drying and demolishing the gastric juices and enzymes in the stomach and as we said earlier the stomach prefers a wet and moist environment and by destroying the gastric juices and enzymes you are destroying the stomach yin whose function is to cool and moisture. If stomach yin is demolished and destroyed there will be stomach heat from an oriental perspective which can lead to stomach ulcers from a western perspective. The more heat there is in the stomach and the more stomach yin is deficient the more inflammation there will be leading to stomach fire from an oriental perspective. This fire will eat the lining of the stomach making the lining thinner and the thinner the lining becomes the weaker the muscular wall of the digestive system will be but particularly the stomach. This weakness in the muscular wall of the stomach will lead to protrusion of the tissue through the weakest part of the muscle and will lead to a condition called Hernia. The function of the spleen is to control muscle tone and strength and when there is a protrusion the spleen is no longer able to hold the organ and tissue in the place where it should be and so it protrudes. In this case, I am only talking about the function of the stomach but generally speaking, you could have Hernia anywhere in the body. Hernia from a western perspective is the protrusion of the muscular tissue of the organ through the weakest point of the muscular wall whether it is Hiatus Hernia or Inguinal Hernia but generally speaking all Hernias are caused by Spleen Qi Deficiency particularly Spleen Yang Deficiency.

2) Yin organ works twenty-four hours a day, Yang organ works when needed

The spleen is a yin organ with a yang job to do. The best way to describe the function of the spleen is to compare it to a pump. The pump is pumping the energy from the sole of the feet up around all of the body for twenty-four hours a day. This represents the venous return of the blood. The stomach is a yang organ with a yin job to do and produces juices most of the time but it will only work when it is required to break down food.

3) Spleen is dense, Stomach is hollow

The spleen is dense, tangible, and material and works for twenty-four hours a day. The stomach is hollow to receive food and mix it with the gastric juices and enzymes and then send it to the small intestine. Most of the digestion process takes place in the small intestine which is the paired organ to the heart. People with Crohn's disease and Ulcerative Colitis will usually have a pale complexion because no nutrients are being extracted by the small intestine. This means the body is losing the nutrients through the digestive process and in this case, there are not enough red blood cells or iron being absorbed by the body and so the person looks pale. The person may also feel tired and exhausted with the slightest effort because they are also not receiving enough oxygen as the red blood cells carry the oxygen. In the case of anemia, it may be due to malfunctioning of a body system or it may be due to the person not eating a well-balanced diet regardless of the reason whether they do not want to gain weight or they have a fear of eating.

4) Spleen energy goes upwards, Stomach energy goes downwards

The spleen energy is equivalent to the heart has to constantly circulate. The function of the spleen is to push up and to hold the organ in the place where it should be. When you breathe in the air goes down and this represents the descending and dispersing function of the lung from an oriental perspective and represents the diffusion from a western aspect. When you eat the food has to go down to the stomach, this is the normal flow of stomach qi and the normal function of stomach qi by blending the food with the gastric juices and enzymes. If a person is poisoned or ate food that did not suit them our job is to divert the stomach qi and not allow the stomach qi to flow in its normal direction. We need to make the stomach qi flow upwards to make the person vomit and to make the spleen qi, especially spleen yang qi, to go downwards to have diarrhea. This is to get rid of the poison from the body before it goes down to blood level. As I described earlier, from an oriental perspective, the practitioner can be thought of as the driver, the needle as the steering wheel, the qi as petrol, and the meridians as the road. Similar to the driver of a car being in charge of what direction the car goes in, the oriental practitioner is in charge of the qi. This means diverting or reversing the flow of qi to make the person achieve their goal by detoxifying the body especially the stomach.

5) Spleen channel and the Stomach channel

The spleen channel begins on the big toe. If a person has Gout, it might affect all of the joints but specifically, it will affect the big toe. This is because the spleen controls the sweet taste and the more protein a person consumes such as eating a lot of red meat and the more sweet food they consume this will lead to the accumulation of uric acid and toxins in the body but especially in the stomach and it will be sent downwards and it will settle in the big toe. One of the things we do to sterilize the big toe is to make it bleed from the point on the side of the nail. We also advise the client to decrease their consumption of protein from the three types of meat, fish, chicken, and particularly red meat. Red meat takes longer for the stomach to digest and we ask people to choose one of the three types of meat and eat only one on the same day. The same applies to sugar and carbohydrate which is a form of sugar. Anything we eat in the final process of digestion will turn into sugar and will be stored in the liver as a form of glycogen and will be released as a form of glucose. We also advise only one type of carbohydrate on the same day.

6) Spleen prefers dryness, Stomach prefers wetness

The stomach contains the gastric juices and the gastric enzymes which are equivalent to the yin whose function is to cool and moisture. The consumption of a lot of greasy oily food will demolish stomach yin and will create internal heat. As I mentioned earlier day is yang and night is yin and the stomach is a yang organ with a yin job to do therefore eating late at night or less than two to three hours before bedtime will damage the stomach function from a structural aspect and will damage its paired organ the spleen from a psychological and emotional aspect. For example, if a person eats a heavy meal late at night and then they try to go to sleep the body will have to deal with two processes at the same time, the physical process of the stomach function trying to digest the food and also the non-physical process of trying to sleep. The physical function of digesting the food is controlled by the brain and the brain is controlled by the sympathetic nervous system which has the function to speed up and create hyperactivity in the body. When we want to go sleep this is a non-physical process related to our heart from an oriental perspective and to our subconscious and mind from a western perspective. The two processes together create a major conflict in the body between the brain, which in this case is responsible for the digestion taking place in the stomach, and your mind which is responsible for taking you to the sleeping and subconscious stage which is the non-physical body.

When you go to sleep you have to pass through four stages:

a) You lie in your bed with your eyes closed but you are still blinking and still breathing normally.

b) The body enters a transitional stage and your eye movements start to decrease and you find it hard to open your eyes or to blink. The physical body gets heavier and the heart rate begins to slow down and body temperature drops.

c) This is one of the most important stages of sleep. The brain and the physical body engage in a battle at this stage between the brain, which is responsible for the demand of the physical body to keep the body alert and awake, and the mind, which is responsible for taking you to the subconscious stage which is opposite to being awake and alert. This stage can be compared to being in a daydream without being asleep. This means your physical body is at rest but your mind is racing and wandering. If your brain and your physical body win the battle against your subconscious and your mind and heart then you will not be able to sleep in the first place. There is another form of insomnia related to yin deficiency where you can fall asleep easily but you wake up during the night and when you wake up you think negative thoughts and create the worst possible scenarios which are not built on reality or facts. If your heart and your subconscious win the battle your brain will no longer be able to respond to the physical demands of your body and you will not feel your body at all.

d) You start to drift very deeply in the sleeping stage. Your senses are decreased. You are closer to your mind and subconscious and you are more attached to your parasympathetic nervous system than to your sympathetic nervous system and the brain. The stronger the detachment between the parasympathetic and sympathetic systems the deeper down the detachment will be to the cellular level and this will determine the state of your sleep and the state of awakening again from your sleep. This is why some people are light sleepers and others are very deep sleepers because the deeper down to the cellular and subconscious level you go the deeper your sleep will be and the weaker your senses will be which is why the deep sleepers don't wake up to noises and you will also wake up refreshed and energized and able to function perfectly the next day.

Physically the brain is in your head and the stomach is in your abdomen. When you eat blood and oxygen have to go down to the stomach and the digestive system to aid the digestive process but yet the location of the brain is in your head and because the blood and oxygen are gone to the digestive system the brain is being deprived of the necessary amount of oxygen to take you to the subconscious stage to go to sleep. Therefore, you are creating a conflict between the two processes, the sleeping related to the subconscious and the digestion related to the stomach.

The consequences of eating late at night are indigestion, heartburn, belching, cramps, spasms, twitching, twisting and turning in bed, and difficulty falling asleep and if you do fall asleep you may have vivid dreams which are due to the interference of the smooth flow of liver qi. The liver controls the ethereal soul, which is responsible for taking you to the state of the subconscious and to have a peaceful night's sleep, and the lungs control the corporeal soul, which is responsible for the state of being alert and awake and controls the physical body which is related to the sympathetic nervous system and the to the brain from a western perspective. To look at it from a western perspective the liver produces enzymes and the gallbladder produces bile, both of these organs aid with digestion, and the function of the bile is to burn fat so if a person eats late at night the body is stimulated to produce bile and so the person will experience the symptoms mentioned above. From an oriental perspective, the energy passes through a channel every two hours and so the state of your mind and the type of dream you will have will also be according to where the energy is flowing.

If you eat your three meals during the day this means your gastric juices have already been used and you do not need to go to bed with your stomach full of heavy food. From a western perspective endorphins, adrenalin and serotonin are hormones responsible for keeping the body in a calm state. If we have a toothache, we could have it at any time of the day or night but mainly the pain will flare up at night because the gastric juices, which are equivalent to the yin and to the endorphins which are the natural painkiller, have been used and this will contribute to being unable to sleep.

If you feel hungry before bed it's recommended you eat very light and easily digestible food that contains fluid and yin such as lettuce, beetroot, or carrot and now below room temperature. The gastric juices represent the yin because they are a form of fluid. A warm drink can also be beneficial before bed along with making time to meditate, slowing your breathing and relaxing your muscles. Avoiding technology, particularly violent programs and social media will help you to have a peaceful night's sleep.

7) Spleen extracts food qi, Stomach receives food qi

The spleen extracts the nutrients from the food we eat. This will depend on what you and how you eat. If you eat a lot of oily and greasy food it will undermine the spleen. Also, anything under room temperature will undermine the spleen from an oriental perspective and the heart from a western perspective because the spleen is equivalent to the heart. Eating a lot of sugary, sweet food will also damage the spleen because the spleen controls the sweet taste. Also, too much carbohydrate will turn to sugar which will turn to a sweet taste. The spleen has to push the energy constantly upwards, which represents the venous return of the heart from a western perspective, and too much sugar, carbohydrate, and protein will accumulate and start to descend and will settle in the lower limbs in the feet but especially in the big toe where the spleen channel begins. This results in an accumulation of sugar, protein, uric acid, and lactic acid. People with Diabetes will have poor and weak circulation, especially in the lower limbs and feet. Diabetes can be described as excess sugar in the blood. If this sugar continues to accumulate and diabetes gets worse, the kidneys will not be able to grip the qi resulting in frequent urination which will further weaken the kidneys. This is why Diabetics feel tired and thirsty because they are already losing fluid. If the spleen does not extract the nutrients you will have a condition called malabsorption and you will see undigested food leaving the body through the body as a form of food. This is an indication of weakness in spleen qi and stomach qi because if the stomach did the job it is supposed to do you would not have undigested food in the stool.

Standing for long periods will also undermine the function of the spleen because it will make the spleen's function of pushing up more difficult and in turn, this will affect digestion. When the spleen extracts the nutrients, it will mix them with air qi (oxygen) to form the Gu qi and the nutritive qi (equivalent to Interstitial fluid) which represents your immune system and the Wei qi (equivalent to the lymphatic system and the immune system).

8) Spleen and Stomach are affected by Damp and Phlegm

Both dampness and phlegm are caused by spleen qi deficiency. Spleen qi deficiency will lead to the accumulation of damp and phlegm. Damp will affect the function of the spleen and generally speaking phlegm affects the function of the stomach. The stomach prefers a wet and moist environment and the spleen prefers a dry environment. Wearing short clothes in damp and windy weather and getting wet will allow dampness to invade the channels particularly the spleen and kidney channel and will affect the function of the channel. Phlegm will invade the stomach and the spleen but will especially affect the stomach and will cause mental confusion, weak memory which worsens in the evening time and a sensation of having a tight band around your forehead. This is called phlegm misting the mind from an oriental perspective. Generally speaking, children with Down syndrome are affected by this condition and sometimes a group of them will share the same signs and symptoms when you check the tongue and the pulse. As I mentioned earlier the spleen from an oriental perspective represents the heart from a western perspective. One of the functions of the heart from an oriental perspective is to capture the mind and help you to sleep. If there is too much phlegm misting the mind it will cause the mind to wander. The physical body will be at rest but because the mind is wandering you will not be able to fall asleep and your mind will start to play tricks on you and give you strange thoughts and ideas. Phlegm from an oriental perspective represents cholesterol from a western perspective which is a waxy substance that blocks the arteries and narrows them. When these arteries are blocked the brain is deprived of oxygen and this affects memory and concentration. Damp descends and will lead to swollen ankles, varicose veins, and weak circulation. Phlegm ascends.

9) Damp and cold undermines the Spleen, Dryness. Heat undermines the Stomach

The stomach prefers a moist environment which is equivalent to the gastric juices and heat will dry moisture and can lead to stomach ulcers. The spleen prefers a dry environment because the spleen energy moves upwards and it is easier to move upwards when there is no obstruction or stagnation such as water. Hence the spleen needs a dry environment to function properly.

High heels make it more difficult for the spleen to function because as I said earlier the spleen represents the heart from a western perspective and the spleen creates the hydraulic pressure to push qi, energy, blood, and fluid back up. From a western perspective, this represents the opening and closing of the valves in your legs. The valves open up to carry blood and then close again. If there is no pressure the blood will accumulate and as the spleen already has to fluid too much wetness will make it more difficult.

10) Damp is heavy and descends downwards

Phlegm is light and moves upwards. Damp is heavy and will cause swelling of the ankles and varicose veins. Phlegm ascends upwards and will cause mental confusion and will affect memory.

11) Damp affects physical activity and strength

Phlegm affects memory and concentration. As we said the spleen controls the physical strength and the state of being tired and exhausted and also controls the extremities especially the lower extremities.

1) Damp is yin, Phlegm is yang
   Damp is yin and descends downwards. Phlegm is yang and ascends upwards.

2) Makes Blood
   The paired yang organ to the spleen is the stomach. If you eat a well-balanced diet the body will have enough nutrients

to extract and to manufacture all that is needed. From a nutrient perspective, the world is built on the five elements and you will need carbohydrates, fats, proteins, vitamins, and fluid. When you have a well-balanced diet, the spleen will extract the nutrients required for the body's systems and organs to function to their optimum level of health and well-being. For people with anorexia and bulimia, the food is gone from the body before the nutrients can be extracted and as the spleen controls the physical strength these people will be weak, tired, and look pale because no food qi is being extracted. Over a long period, this will lead to anemia and in turn will damage the stomach qi. If you don't eat there will be no new blood manufactured hence the reason for looking pale.

3) Holds Qi in place

The spleen holds the qi and the organs in place. The blood is regarded as an organ from an oriental perspective. Blood is yin in nature and qi is yang in nature. When spleen Qi is strong the muscles will be strong especially in the lower limbs and the blood will be held in the veins and arteries and will not leak out. If a person sits or stands for long periods it will lead to spleen qi deficiency and may cause varicose veins. Standing for long periods will undermine the spleen and will affect the venous return of the blood and will lead to varicose veins due to spleen qi deficiency but especially spleen yang deficiency. Too much sitting means that qi is stagnant and may lead to hemorrhoids. From an oriental perspective when a tissue or organ protrudes (leaks out of place) it is due to spleen qi stagnation, the qi is not moving.

4) Controls the muscles

The spleen controls the muscular system. The strength, power, flexibility, and tone of your muscles are determined by spleen qi. If the spleen qi is weakened or deficient, physical and muscular strength will get weaker. The weakness in muscles will lead to a hernia, a protrusion of the tissue and the organ from the weakest point regardless of where it is located, such as hiatus hernia or inguinal hernia. Another example is in the case of a stroke. There are two types of stroke, the first stroke caused by a clot and the second is a stroke caused by an aneurysm when the blood leaks through a weakened point in the artery and veins when the artery bursts. This is caused by spleen qi deficiency from an oriental perspective. Veins and arteries are muscular tubes and the blood has to stay flowing inside the veins and arteries and should not leak and cause a clot. If we trace back the deficiency of the spleen from a channel perspective, we will see the deterioration of the functional aspect of the spleen. What I mean by this is, the spleen channel starts on the side of the big toe and the dysfunction of this area leads to gout, calcification, bunion, and build-up of lactic acid, further up the channel the deterioration is varicose veins, further up again will be hemorrhoids, further up again will be a hernia and the highest will be an aneurysm. You will notice that there are five locations relating to the five elements. From an oriental perspective, any health problem related to the function of our limb circulation, core, and lower back will represent the functional aspect of the spleen.

5) Short Term Memory

As I mentioned earlier, we have two types of memory. The long-term memory represents your past is related to the kidneys and represents your DNA from an oriental perspective. DNA is the genetic material you inherited from your parents at the time of conception. This will be explained in further detail when we discuss the kidneys.

Short term memory is related to your spleen from an oriental perspective and represents the present moment and the now. As we now know the spleen represents your physical strength which represents the state of being tired or exhausted or being strong or energized because the spleen is the only organ that has to keep pushing the energy from the toes up to the head even while you are asleep. This explains why if you are overtired or exhausted it will affect your short-term memory. When you are overtired you start to do silly things and forget the slightest thing. If this state of exhaustion lasts for a long period without giving the body enough rest to rejuvenate and recover it will start to affect the state of your mind and as we know the represents the heart and this means that your mind will not be captured and you will be in a state similar to a daydream, you will find yourself becoming forgetful. If the deterioration continues it makes the person form scenarios in their head. These scenarios are delusional and not based on reality, for example, going to check the door over and over to check if it locked and even though each time you check the door it is locked you keep going back to check it again. From an oriental perspective drinking a lot of water and eating a well-balanced diet containing omega oil will help to restore and improve your memory. Activities such as swimming, cycling, reading, and visualizing scenes will also help to restore your emotional state and wellbeing, but especially to the state of your hormones. This is why in women, the memory will be affected at the time of the period, ovulation and menopause because the hormonal imbalance leads to a chemical balance. In turn, this chemical imbalance will affect all processes, in particular emotional, behavioural, and psychological processes. These processes are not related to your anatomy and physiologies because they are not related to a specific organ for example memory, focus, concentration, intuition, wisdom, and perception. All of these are related to the state of your mind and the state of your psychological feelings.

If you have anaemia this will affect both types of memory but particularly the short-term memory because when an anaemic body is lacking in iron it will be lacking in red blood cells whose job is to carry oxygen to all the systems and organs in the body and especially to the brain. In this case, the brain is deprived of the sufficient amount of oxygen, blood supply and fluid needed and this will affect your memory. If you are anaemic i.e. not eating enough iron, the spleen has nothing to extract and because the spleen controls the physical strength, power and extremities you will feel tired, in turn, this will affect your memory. If you are anaemic and your body is lacking in iron and oxygen this will affect the quantity and quality and composition of the blood. The function of the blood from an oriental perspective is to capture the mind and if the mind is not captured it will be wandering and will not be in the present moment for example when a person is talking to you but their mind is engaged elsewhere. The state of your mind will determine the state of your memory and the state of your memory will determine the state of your mind. Both your mind and your memory are related to the state of your emotional feelings and from an oriental perspective, a physical complaint will become an emotional complaint and likewise become a physical complaint.

Generally speaking, from an oriental perspective there is individual memory and collective memory like there is individual karma and collective karma.

Individual Memory

We don't know if we inherit memory or not but we know that the memory we have depends on the state of our parent's mind and health. Psychological and emotional problems are not contagious and if a mother has depression it does not mean that her baby will be born with depression. Our memory will be influenced by the way we are brought up. The way we are brought up will establish and create psychological and behavioural problems. If a mother and father are depressed and their newborn baby is not, the baby will develop depression through the process of learned behaviour from the way parents think and act, in turn this will affect the baby's memory.

Collective memory is best explained using an example. If you have one class with ten students who are weak at mathematics the best way to improve the weaker students is to mix them with the stronger students to create a balance between the yin and yang. The collective stimulation of the human intellect starts as a baby through their upbringing. This explains why sometimes you will see parents who are very strong and good at mathematics and this might pass to their children through the collective karma. Another example is doctors whose children also become doctors. This is also due to the support and encouragement the parents give to their children and it will help the child's intellect and their sense of direction in life in general particularly in their career and their career choices. Regardless of what they want to be the child will need a good memory, focus, and concentration along with a good level of intellect and mental capacity which will be influenced by the collective karma I am talking about.

Spleen from a Five Element Perspective

According to the five elements the spleen represents the earth because it is in the middle of Jiao. Taste the spleen controls the sweet taste. The spleen is equivalent to the function of the heart and the pancreas from a western perspective. The function of the pancreas is to produce insulin to control the amount of sugar being circulated by the heart through the body creating a tiny network called capillaries. Because the spleen has to push energy twenty-four hours a day and controls the sweet taste if a person eats a lot of food, carbohydrates, or protein it will lead to calcification and gout and as we now know if we have gout we will have it in the big toe because this is where the spleen channel starts. Also, people with diabetes will have weak and poor circulation, especially in their feet. This is because of the malfunction of the spleen from an oriental perspective and because of excessive consumption of sugar which goes to the spleen through its paired organ the stomach. When you consume a lot of sweet foods or fizzy drinks this will affect the spleen function by creating false and extreme energy and you will feel very energized or hyper and then all of a sudden you will start to feel very lethargic and weak. In some cases because the blood sugar ruses and declines so rapidly it will make the person feel very sleepy and sometimes they will sleep immediately after eating. This is called 'false energy' because it is released at once and it is diminished at once. This sort of energy will have no chance to be stored, unlike the sugar and energy you have after eating rice, potato, pasta, or bread which in the final process of digestion will turn to sugar and will be stored in the liver as a form of glycogen. The difference is that this type of energy will be released only when it is required and it will be released at a very gradual and slow pace. Either way, when the person stops eating or they fast or go on a diet the body starts to use what it has stored in it. The body is designed to release energy from rice, potato, pasta, bread, etc. gradually but the body is not able to release energy from fizzy drinks gradually, instead it will increase the energy in one shot and decrease it in one shot which creates a state of imbalance in all of the body but especially in the digestive and muscular system. As I mentioned earlier our main job is to restore balance because that's what our medicine is all about, balancing the yin with the yang.

Colour

The spleen represents the colour yellow from a five-element point of view Direction Centre represents the direction of the spleen because the earth is the centre between the sun and the moon. The digestive system is in the middle portion of the viscera between the vascular, respiratory, reproduction, and excretory systems.

Sound

The sound related to the spleen from a five-element perspective is neutral.

CHAPTER 8

PATTERNS OF THE SPLEEN

Generally speaking, the Spleen is one of the most important organs from an oriental perspective. Before we talk about the spleen as an organ and as a channel it is important to clarify something: the spleen is one of the most important organs from an oriental perspective, we don't mean the structural aspect of the spleen which is related to our anatomy and physiology. What we mean is the functional aspect of the spleen as a yin organ and the functional aspect of the spleen channel as a yin channel. The function of the spleen from an oriental perspective is similar and equivalent to the function of the heart from a western perspective. For example, if you have a flat tyre you need to put air in the tyre, the pumping action of putting the air in the tyre will lift the tyre off the ground and the tyre will no longer be flat. The spleen does the same by acting as a pump for twenty-four hours, even while you are asleep, to pump the blood back to the heart from the sole of the feet and the toes. This action is done by the spleen by holding the qi, blood and fluid and keeping them flowing inside the veins, arteries and capillaries while returning the blood to the heart and lungs to be oxygenated again for the circulation to start all over again. The blood leaves our heart from the left side and descends, with the direction of gravity. This is why spleen qi has to be very strong, especially spleen yang qi which has the function of holding the organ and tissue in place where they should be to push the blood back up against gravity. As I mentioned earlier, from an oriental perspective blood is considered as an organ. The blood has to be held inside the vessels, veins, arteries and capillaries until it returns to the heart without any leakages in any place or at any stage during the circulation. This all depends on the functional aspect of the spleen, especially spleen qi and the spleen yang qi. Qi is yang in nature and blood and yin is in nature, blood nourishes qi and qi has to be very strong, especially yang qi, to push the blood forcefully back to the heart for the circulation process to start again. The movement of the blood back to the heart represents the venous return of deoxygenated blood from a western perspective and an anatomy and physiology point of view. This is why from an oriental perspective we say that the spleen represents the heart from a western perspective. The heart is a yin organ and has a yang job to do which is to constantly pump and circulate the blood around the body's tissues and organs down to the cellular level. The pumping action of the heart represents the yang aspect and as we now know yang is activity and movement. The spleen is a yin organ and a yin channel but it has a yang job to do and has to constantly hold organs in place. The spleen channel starts from the medial side of the big toe and goes upwards which means the direction of flow of spleen energy from a functional aspect is yang in nature.

Spleen Qi Deficiency

This condition is caused by irregular eating habits, excessive mental strain and thinking, by chronic illness or chronic use of medications.

1) Irregular eating habits

Irregular eating habits come under the category of the following: What you eat, When you eat and How you eat.

Eating late at night cause spleen qi deficiency and damages the stomachs gastric juices which are equivalent to the yin from an oriental perspective and has the job of cooling and moistening the stomach. The reason for spleen qi becoming deficient by eating late at night is because daytime is yang and night is yin and when you eat your three meals during the day you have your gastric juices that were produced by the process of digestion. When the gastric juices have been already used anything you eat in the night-time, especially a heavy meal with hot spicy and greasy food, will lead to spleen qi deficiency and stomach qi deficiency and you will have the following symptoms: Indigestion, Heartburn, Hiccup, Belching and burping, Passing Wind.

All of these symptoms will interfere with the quality and quantity of your sleep when you go to bed at night and you will find it difficult to find a comfortable position in bed. This will affect your breathing because you are creating an internal conflict between your mind, which is responsible for taking you to the subconscious stage to sleep, and your physical body which is responsible for starting the digestion process for the food you ate. Your brain is in your head, the upper part of your body, and your stomach is in the middle part of your body. To initiate the sleeping process the brain needs enough oxygen for the mind to enter the subconscious stage which is necessary to start the sleeping process in the first place. This oxygen is carried by the circulation of the heart but when you eat late at night your stomach and digestive system also need the oxygen which is also carried by the blood to start the digestive process.

When you eat late at night you not only cause spleen qi deficiency or stomach qi deficiency you are also causing huge conflicts inside your body:

1. Structural conflict:

The first conflict is structural and is related to anatomy and physiology. This structural conflict will affect the heart as an organ and the vascular as a system. What I mean is instead of the blood being pumped and focusing energy, fluid and oxygen on the brain to start the sleeping process, instead, the blood will be pumped down to the stomach to start the digestive process. This creates a major conflict between the functional aspect of the flow of qi, blood and oxygen especially the spleen qi and stomach qi.

2. Emotional conflict:

The emotional conflict will be created when you eat late at night. This is another reason for the spleen qi to become deficient. This conflict is caused by the following:

A) Sympathetic system is to speed up and is yang in nature. It is linked and connected to our physical body from a functional, anatomical and physiology perspective.

The digestive process will activate our sympathetic nerve system every time we eat by the starting of peristalsis action which is a series of wave-like muscle contractions that move food through the digestive tract. The pancreas starts the release of the insulin to control the amount of sugar that's being pumped into the bloodstream every time you eat. When you eat your blood sugar rises especially when you eat carbohydrates or sweet food. This will create a state of hyperactivity as the overstimulation of the brain and sympathetic nerve system and because the huge amount of glucose will be pumped suddenly to the brain. This state of hyperactivity is opposite to the state that you need before you go to bed to sleep.

The heart has to capture the mind for the person who is trying to sleep to enter the subconscious state. The capturing of the mind by the heart is a non-physical, non-tangible and non-substantial process however the heart is now doing a physical process which is carrying the blood down to the stomach to start the digestive process which starts a major conflict between the subconscious and the conscious from an oriental perspective and a battle between the sympathetic and the parasympathetic from a western perspective and an anatomy and physiology point of view. You should not eat at least two hours before going to bed and if you feel hungry you could eat a light type of food such as cucumber, lettuce or salad which is yin in nature and will cool and nourish. Honey acts as a sedative and can be taken before going to bed. The more yin you have the more peaceful your night's sleep will be. People who work night shifts will often ask what they should do to help them to sleep. If they finish work at 8 a.m. then they should stop eating two hours beforehand which would be 6 a.m.

What you eat

This is another reason that leads to spleen qi and stomach qi deficiency. Anything you eat and put in your mouth will have an effect on your body and your health in general but especially on the digestive as a system and the stomach and spleen as organs.

Sugar

Consuming too much sugar and sweet foods will lead to diabetes. Diabetes will damage the sight as a sense and will also damage the circulation. The worse the circulation is the more the limbs will be deprived of oxygen and nutrients. People with diabetes have very poor circulation and in some cases, they lose the sensation in their lower limbs and feet due to death of the tissue. This situation declares the start of gangrene.

Not consuming enough sugar results in hypoglycaemia. The person will feel tired and exhausted with the slightest effort or from doing nothing at all. This will indicate the severity of the condition.

Hypoglycaemia, low blood pressure and ME (chronic fatigue syndrome) will all affect our immune system. Low blood pressure indicates the weakness of the immune system, muscular system and the skin. From an oriental perspective, the skin and the muscles are part of the immune system which is in the first barrier of defence.

The Wei qi represents the immune and lymphatic system. When the weather is cold the skin pores close, the hairs stand up to preserve heat, the muscles shrink and the blood will be taken away from your limbs to supply and concentrate on your organs. This is part of the body's defensive mechanism which is one of the functions of our immune and lymphatic system, to protect us against the pathogenic invaders such as bacteria and viruses and to prevent them entering from the exterior environment to the interior environment and from attacking our body tissues and organs down to cellular level. The same principle can be applied to ME and hypoglycaemia. The only exception with ME is the bacteria and viruses, which are the pathogenic invaders, are residual in all our respiratory system in general but especially in the lungs. The invaders are ready to flare up at any time and this depends on your lifestyle especially your emotional state and the state how you are feeling. To look at it from a western perspective it is the same, when you go to your GP and they tell you that you are run down your immune system will be weak because the more stress you are under the weaker your immune system will be.

Protein

Consuming too much protein leads to gout and the build-up of calcification of uric and lactic acid and protein in all of the body's joints but especially the big toe because the spleen channel starts on the big toe and the channel will be blocked from the start. A bunion is a calcification, it is very thick with rough skin and can be either on the ball of the feet or beside it or can manifest as cracked and painful heels. The reason for this is because on the medial side you have the kidney and on the lateral side you have the urinary bladder if you have too much protein your urine will be yellow and strong and will smell because the kidneys are not able to cope.

Too little protein means there is no energy because the protein forms the energy block for your physical activity and physical strength. It can be compared to cement used for a building; you cannot build the building without cement.

Salt

Too much salt leads to high blood pressure. Too little salt leads to low blood pressure. Generally speaking, any condition related to deficiency is better than excess. For example, it is better to have diarrhoea than to have constipation, yet both are not normal to have. However, with the diarrhoea, your immune system, lungs and respiratory system are not strong enough to push the toxins out of the body. Having high blood pressure can lead to stroke which subsequently leads to paralysis. Having low blood pressure could be rectified by going to the root cause of the problem which could be, for example, not having enough salt in your diet.

When a woman's period is long it means the body can cleanse itself. The period means the body is taking an internal shower and washing from the inside. It is always easy to treat the deficiency by adding to the body what it lacks in the first place. For example, if a person is anaemic due to a lack of iron you can ask them to eat red meat with no fat in it and also eat a lot of green vegetables or take an iron tablet. Any excess condition is much more difficult to treat because it is usually due to a build-up over years and years and did not happen overnight. Let me clarify something, not always the excess is related to your diet or to what you eat, sometimes the excess is produced and manufactured by your body. For example, a vegetarian could have high cholesterol and also their iron level could be high and as we said too much iron will affect the eyesight. Our job is to create the balance from every aspect and in this case from a nutrient aspect.

Calcium

Too much calcium is not good because it is regarded as an excess condition which causes the heart to have an irregular heartbeat. For a long period, it will damage the heart and the valves from an anatomy and physiology perspective. Too much calcium also causes a lot of phlegm, mucus and damp and fluid to form which in return will block your sinus and your nose. The sinus is the first gate to the respiratory system and when the sinus is blocked, the respiratory system will pay the price. Muscular contraction needs calcium, potassium, magnesium and sodium and the heart is a muscle. If you run you will sweat and you lose sodium and get cramps. Too much calcium is another form of cramp and contraction. Too little calcium or no calcium will lead to brittle bones and a weak skeletal system and osteoporosis.

Iron

Too much iron leads to hemochromatosis. Eventually, excess iron will affect the sight and will lead to cramp, spasm, tightness and stiffness in all of the joints but especially the hips and ankle. From an oriental perspective, the reason is that the gallbladder channel starts on the ankle and goes to the hip on the side of the leg. The liver is yin and gallbladder is yang and both channels are put under massive pressure because of the excess iron. Excess iron will also lead to constipation.

Too little iron leads to anaemia. When there is not enough iron it means there is not enough haemoglobin (not enough oxygen) and this is why people with anaemia feel tired, because there is not enough oxygen. Anaemia for a long period will also lead to constipation, because the blood is regarded as a yin organ and the function of the blood is to cool and moisten and due to the anaemia, there is nothing to cool and moisten, especially in the bowel. To link with western medicine, the function of the lungs is to take oxygen (air qi) from the external environment and descend the oxygen to its paired organ the large intestine. This means there is not enough oxygen or fluid being descended by the function of the lungs which control the descending and dispersing to the bowel. In return, this will lead to constipation. Constipation is a sign of dryness and because the lungs control the skin the skin will become dry also.

The lack of oxygen, haemoglobin and iron will cause weakness of lung qi and will affect the descending and dispersing function of the lungs. Dispersing from an oriental perspective represents the diffusion from a western perspective and descending aids the process of defecation. It is a vicious circle because when the yin organ is affected its paired yang organ will pay the price and vice versa. Generally speaking, the dryness will affect the large intestine as a channel and as an organ and will affect the stomach as a channel and as an organ.

Generally speaking, when people have too much iron it is not always related to their diet. Unfortunately, sometimes our body can produce too much iron. This can be seen in people who are vegetarian but their iron and cholesterol levels are high. On the contrary, a person might eat a lot of red meat and their cholesterol could be perfect. In this case, we ask the person to do the following:

- Drink a lot of water especially water that does not contain fluoride and chloride such as the filtered water.
- People with too much iron should avoid eating a lot of red meat and green vegetables. They should also avoid eating vitamin C because vitamin C helps the absorption of iron.
- Drink a lot of strong tea and strong coffee because in this case, we don't want the body to absorb the iron. Drinking decaffeinated tea or coffee is not good for the body because the substances used to make the tea or coffee decaffeinated will have a huge impact on the body in general but especially on the liver which has the function of detoxifying and cleansing the body.

Fat

Too much fat will lead to cholesterol, Cholesterol leads to arteriosclerosis which is a hardening of the interior wall of the artery. For a long period, this will lead to a blockage and in return, it will lead to a heart attack. Generally speaking, from an oriental perspective any medical condition will have two types, for example, yin asthma and yang asthma, yin headache and yang headache, yin heart attack when the tongue drops to the right and yang heart attack when the tongue drops to the left. Even from a western perspective sometimes when a person has a heart attack there are no symptoms because the blockage, in this case, is not in the aorta instead the blockage might be in the branches of the vascular system like the capillaries. That's what people mean why they say someone had a massive heart attack, it means the aorta and the heart itself is affected immediately.

The same rule applies when a person is vegetarian and their cholesterol is high. The person might eat a lot of oily, greasy, fatty food but their cholesterol is perfect. From both an oriental and a western perspective is we have good fat and bad fat. The good fat is the fat you get from olive oil, fish, omega oils, etc. The bad fat is gotten from animal fat. Regardless of the reason why, whether fat is created by our body or ingested from foods our job is to create the balance by telling the person to avoid too much oily greasy, fatty, raw food, avoid eating or drinking anything below room temperature and do a lot of cardiovascular exercises to increase heartbeat, create heat and sweat.

From an oriental perspective, we tonify the gallbladder because the function of the gallbladder is to burn the fat. Too little fat will affect our memory, concentration, focus and intellect. If you do not have enough fat you will start to forget, especially your short-term memory. The brain needs fat for memory, concentration and focus. If you steam and boil your food for a long period and don't eat any fat you will start to see the decline of your memory and the weakness of your circulation and you will also start to feel colder than usual. The function of the fat is to provide warmth and to also provide protection to our internal organs against any injury or accident. From an oriental perspective if a person has too much fat in their body it is better to turn it into muscle rather than losing it. This is why we do not agree with every person who comes to the clinic that they need to lose weight. The reason for this is because you need to have at least 10kg of extra fat in your body because when you get sick the body starts to depend on its storage. The general rule, whether from an oriental perspective or western perspective is if your height is 180 and you subtract 100 then 80 is left, this is your perfect balance in relation to your height but it is not the perfect balance for your health as you have no extra to fall on and you have to have extra.

How you eat

How you eat will be another reason that causes spleen qi deficiency. What we mean by how you eat from an oriental perspective is the following.

• Do you chew your food enough? The longer you chew the food in your mouth the less work the stomach has to do. This means chewing the food will play major role in the digestive process from the beginning to the end. If you don't chew your food enough it will damage the gastric juices and gastric enzymes and will lead to the following: indigestion, belching, heartburn, hiccups, flatulence, bloating and acid reflux. We can determine if the condition is excess of deficiency by asking the client if they feel better after passing wind. If the answer is yes then the condition is excess as they feel better after releasing it even for a short while. If the answer is no the condition is deficiency. In relation to excess or deficiency, from a physical aspect if you have a headache or any form of pain and you put your hand on the sore spot and the pain eases it is deficiency. If you put your hand on the sore spot and the pain gets worse it is excess.

• The saliva in your mouth produces enzymes. These enzymes aid the digestive process and in return makes the stomachs' job much easier as it has to work less and produce less gastric juice. As we said earlier the stomachs gastric juices are yin in nature because their job is to break down the food which is received by the mouth into the oesophagus through a process called peristalsis which is the muscular contraction of the digestive tract to squeeze and push the food down from the mouth into the stomach. From a western perspective this process of swallowing the food after being chewed in the mouth is done with the coordination of the nerve system and muscular system. If the nerve that triggers the contraction of the digestive tract is damaged due to an injury or due to a stroke or heart attack the swallowing process either becomes very slow and difficult or it becomes impaired altogether. In a very severe case, the person's sense of taste and speech will be affected because your taste bud will be affected and because from an oriental perspective the tongue opens into the heart and so the speech will be affected also.

• If a person eats a lot of food which is yin in nature and contains a lot of fluid and moisture such as lettuce, cucumber or watermelon, this will help the stomach and will help the gastric juices and gastric enzymes by improving their functioning aspect. It is completely the opposite if a person eats a lot of hot and spicy or oily greasy food or a lot of red meat as this will damage the gastric enzymes and gastric juices because this type of food is yang in nature. In this case the yang will consume the yin and the gastric enzymes will be decreased and demolished because this food will lead to heat and dryness and this heat over a long period of time will weaken the internal tissue and erode it. In return this will lead to an ulcer and the deeper the ulcer descends down the more protrusion we will have and the more leakage we will have. Both the ulcer and the hernia are caused by spleen qi deficiency but the difference between them is the hernia is defined as the protrusion of the internal tissue through the weakest points of the muscle for example a hiatus hernia. With an ulcer there is also protrusion and erosion but in this case it protrudes the part that is already eroded. In the worst scenario the person might have both an ulcer and a hernia at the same time. Eating a lot of red meat and drinking a lot of alcohol will lead to constipation and sometimes can also lead to diarrhoea. This depends on what type of heat you have, empty heat or excess heat. Generally speaking, both the stomach and the bowel prefer a wet and moist environment and the spleen prefers a dry environment. The small intestine and the large intestine need to be at a certain temperature in order for them to function correctly. Any decrease or increase in the internal temperature whether caused by eating a lot of spicy food or cold, raw or freezing food or drinking dirty water as a result of food poisoning will interfere with the process of digestion and excretion.

• Eating standing up. This will interfere with the spleens function of extracting the Gu qi (food qi). From both an oriental perspective and western perspective it will interfere with the function of extracting the nutrients and minerals from the food and drink. Eating standing up. Eating fast or in a hurry and drinking any form of liquid which is below room temperature will all lead to spleen qi deficiency but especially spleen yang deficiency and stomach yin deficiency and this will affect all the digestive system from a structural and functional aspect.

Deficiency/Excess:

To locate the ovaries, go four fingers to the side from the bellybutton and from that point go four fingers down. This will be the location of the ovaries on each side. If the woman finds the ovaries during the time of their period or ovulation, they will feel a difference between the two sides. One side will be tenderer than the other and the pulse will be stronger when you breathe in and out. Liver qi goes around the reproductive system to start the period. If there is a blockage the liver qi keeps pushing qi to start the period and you will get throbbing. This also depends on the emotional state the woman is in at the time and the state of their mind because this will interfere with the smooth flow of qi and will interfere with the process of starting and stopping the period and the process of ovulation and in some cases will interfere with the fertility. This is why the woman is able to have her first child and she is not able to have her second child, this is called secondary fertility from a western perspective. You will find that parents are so desperate and eager to have a baby and as soon as they go to adopt the woman will get pregnant. The reason for this the aspect of letting go whether from an emotional or physical aspect will help all of our body's systems and organs from a structural and function aspect down to cellular level.

3. Excessive mental strain and excessive mental thinking

As we said earlier when we were talking about the function of the spleen from an oriental perspective one of the functions is to control our muscles and extremities especially our legs. In return our muscles control our physical constitution and control our physical strength. Another one of the spleens functions is to control our short-term memory which is related to the present moment. This memory is linked and connected to our daily activity. What we mean by excessive mental strain is an excessive way of thinking especially in a negative, worrying and pessimistic way. This is will destroy our spleen qi and our mind and in return will affect our short-term memory. The state of our mind and short-term memory are both linked and connected to the state of our physical strength. Physical strength is opposite to the state of being tired and exhausted. This means you are being refreshed and energised and full of life and energy and are able to do your daily activities. An excessive way of thinking will put the spleen under huge strain and in return this strain will affect our physical strength and physical energy. This is why people who deal with figures for a long period of time, such as an accountant, will feel more tired and exhausted when they finish work than the people who do physical work such as builders. Both of them are burning calories when they are working but the calories the accountant is burning are not physical calories related to our anatomy and physiology instead, they are related to the state of mind and state of focus, concentration, intellect and mental capacity. All of these depend on the state of your mind and memory, especially the short-term memory which is linked and directly connected to your spleen. For example, consider the following experiment, you give John a glass and a towel and ask him to keep running up and down the length of a hall, you tell him when he starts to sweat to wipe his face with the towel and squeeze the sweat from the towel into the glass. John does this and when we take the glass and put it on the scale to measure the amount of sweat produced, we see that John burned 100 calories. These calories are physical calories and are related and produced by the activity of John's body, the physical body. However, when a person thinks they are also burning calories but these are not physical, material or substantial calories. They are not produced by our physical body or by the body's activity; instead they are produced by the state of our mind and the state of our subconscious. This means the power of your mind and the power of your subconscious will determine the amount of calories you produce at the time when you are thinking whether in a positive or negative way. Generally speaking, the negative way of thinking will cause more damage and have more of an impact and effect on our mind and subconscious than the positive way of thinking. The reason for this is karma. Consider working with someone for nine hours a day and they are doom and gloom compared to working with someone nine hours a day and they are positive. The emotional calories will cause more damage and will have a destructive effect on our health, mind and memory more so than the physical calories. The physical exhaustion and physical tiredness which makes you produce physical calories to do your job could be dealt with and managed in a very easy and simple physical way. In the earlier example when John was running, he felt very tired after it and you told him to go and have a bath and a rest, the next day John tells you he feels more energised and doesn't feel tired and exhausted any more. In this case the bath and rest helped John. However, the problem with the emotional calories in that the human produces and burns them when they are thinking and we cannot apply the same principle to the exhaustion and tiredness that we applied when John was tired from running. If you are thinking so deeply, especially in a worried and anxious way about something and you have certain emotion that is affecting how you think then this will make you feel very drained and exhausted and as you say 'on the verge of having a nervous breakdown'. Regardless of what these emotions are at the time the person is thinking we cannot tell them to go to sleep and when you wake up you will not feel angry or sadness or worried and everything will be fine. Unfortunately, it doesn't work like that. That is what I mean when I say the difference between physical calories and emotional calories. Emotional calories have more of an impact and damage on our health and that is excessive mental strain damages the body more than the physical work.

Let me give you another example, when you drive your car on a long journey you will feel tired and exhausted. If you want to look at it from an anatomy and physiology perspective you are not doing any physical activity that causes your heart rate and circulation to speed up. In this case from an oriental perspective is what makes you feel tired if you are not doing any physical activity? The answer is the overwork by the spleen to keep your mind, focus and concentration and all your senses at the highest state of alertness so that you will not have a car accident. This will take its toll on the physical body and makes the body feel tired and exhausted and in return this will have its effect on your mind and on your subconscious and on your memory, especially your short-term memory. This is why when you are tired you start to notice a decline in your concentration, focus and short term memory and you start to make silly mistakes and forget things like forgetting where you left your keys or reading a newspaper and forgetting the first line before reading the second line. From a personal experience I see it when I am coaching the local junior football team, when the players get tired and exhausted, they start to make a lot of silly mistakes like passing the ball and giving to back to the opponent without being under any form of pressure, their judgement will also be affected and they choose the wrong option when they have the ball or instead of passing the ball the player shoots.

Whether the mind is under strain or the body is under strain both of them will cause spleen qi deficiency whether you look at it from an oriental perspective or western perspective. Our job is to tonify the spleen and create balance with its paired organ the stomach and to create balance in all the body from every aspect. This is what oriental medicine is all about, balancing the yin with the yang.

4. Chronic disease and illness and chronic use of medications for long periods of time

Generally speaking, any chronic disease and illness will have an effect and impact on the persons health in general but the affected organ will especially pay the price more.

As we know, smoking affects all of our health in general but the lungs and the respiratory will pay the price more. Drinking alcohol will affect all of the body but the liver will pay the price more. If you eat a lot of spicy food the stomach and the spleen will pay the price.

What makes matters worse is if the chronic disease is combined with the usage of medications for long periods of time.

For example, long time use of an inhaler will damage the lungs, cortisone and steroid creams will damage the skin, and medications for headaches will damage the lining of the intestines and the stomach. From an oriental perspective any usage of drugs and medicines for long periods of time will demolish and damage the yin in general but especially the yin of the affected organ directly. As you know the function of the yin is to cool and moisten the body's systems, organs and tissues down to cellular level. The use of medications will demolish stomach yin which is demolishing the gastric juices and gastric enzymes from a western perspective. The stronger the medication and the larger the dosage, especially over a long period of time, the more yin that will be demolished and the yin of all of the body will dry up because there is now nothing left to cool and moisten the organs and the internal tissue. This will result in the lining of the stomach getting thinner which can sometimes lead to a stomach ulcer and to internal bleeding or hernia. From a western medical perspective the same theory will be applied because the use of medications for long periods of time will weaken all of our body in general but especially the immune system. The reason for this is because using the medications for long periods of time results in the body becoming immune to them. For example, using a lot of antibiotics in a short period of time will have an adverse effect on our body and on our health in general. A doctor will usually prescribe antibiotics depending on the following:

> ➢ What type of bacteria is invading your body and immune system
> ➢ How serious the condition is
> ➢ How weak or how strong your immune system was before the illness because there are a variety of reasons that makes

our immune system weak and that make us susceptible to a lot of illnesses especially colds and flu. Some of these reasons:

➢ Poor diet. A balanced diet should contain carbohydrates, proteins, fat, vitamins and minerals and fluids. These make up the 5 elements.

➢ Not having enough rest or sleep. When we sleep at night our body goes through a process of rejuvenating itself.

➢ Anaemia and low iron levels will affect our immune systems.

➢ Drinking alcohol

➢ Smoking

➢ Eating pork or a lot of red meat

➢ Stress, anxiety and worrying have a great deal of impact on the immune system and on our health in general. The main sign that your immune system is being affected by stress and anxiety is when you start to have mouth ulcers and a low energy level. Your memory will also be affected because your mind will not be grounded and it will be distracted very easily. In return this will affect our memory, focus and concentration especially our short-term memory which is linked to our spleen as an organ and our spleen as a channel from an oriental perspective.

➢ Dehydration. Seventy per cent of our body is made up of water and dehydration can weaken our immune system. Later I will talk more about dehydration and water.

Sometimes after finishing a course of antibiotics you will find that you need another stronger course of antibiotics. This indicates the weakness of your immune system and the strength of the pathogenic invader that has attacked your body and immune system and in turn will lead to spleen qi deficiency and will affect all of the body but especially it's paired organ the stomach.

The person who has spleen qi deficiency will have the following signs and symptoms:

1. Pale complexion

Spleen qi deficiency affects the function of the spleen which is extracting the nutrients of the food to make blood. From a western perspective this condition is known as malabsorption where the body is not able to finish the digestive process fully. Hence the body is not able to extract enough calories required from the food eaten. One of the signs of malabsorption is undigested food in the bowel movement. From an oriental perspective this indicates weakness of spleen and stomach qi and also weakness of the digestive system in general. Another example is ulcerative colitis or Crohn's disease where undigested food can be seen in the bowel movement along with blood. When there is not enough blood the person will look pale.

2. Anorexia, weak stomach qi, distension, bloating

Anxiety and worry weaken the stomach and spleen qi. This weakness will lead to rebellious stomach qi. This means instead of food going downward it goes upward. Sometimes this can happen naturally due to the weakness of the stomach and spleen qi and sometimes the weakness is caused by the use of strong medications such as antibiotics which causes the person to vomit. This condition can sometimes be self-inflicted by the person who has spleen qi deficiency. The best example of this is the person who has bulimia or anorexia. The main reason for these illnesses are either emotional or psychological which means the problem is related to the persons behaviour more than their physical constitution. What I mean by this is the person will behave according to the way how they think and the way how they view themselves. In the case of bulimia or anorexia when the person looks in the mirror, they think that they are fat even though they thin, this is what makes them make themselves vomit and therefore not keeping the nutrients in the body. Sometimes these people will have low self-esteem and lack of confidence and self-belief and will be easily led and influenced by the collective mind of the society. Society puts a lot of pressure on us about our image and how we should look, people with bulimia and anorexia use their collective mind and don't use their individual mind, instead they want to please society with the way they look more than they want to please themselves. They will also want to show a happy and smiley face to the public and sometimes they like having inappropriate conversations. However, the problem is that the way you think will become the way you feel and the way you feel will become the way you think and behave. From a Muslim perspective this is not always the case because the way you look does not represent the way you feel and the way you feel does not represent how you look. You might look like you are wealthy and have nice clothes but you are miserable and sad and vice versa. Sometimes when people make themselves vomit it is caused by the environment they live in and that they are surrounded by. For example, if you live with a dominating mother or father who tries to control your life you will try to rebel against them and the only choice and decision you are in charge of is making yourself vomit. This means your mind will be rebellious. A rebellious mind will lead to rebellious behaviour and rebellious behaviour will affect and impact all of our body but in this case, it will affect our spleen and stomach and that is why you have spleen qi deficiency and rebellious spleen qi and stomach qi.

3. Loose stool, oedema, and swollen lower limbs

One of the spleens functions is to push everything back to the heart again such as the fluid, blood, lymph, etc. This depends on the yang function aspect of the spleen. If there is spleen qi deficiency and spleen yang deficiency the fluid will not descend up and will result in the swollen lower limbs especially the ankles and because spleen yang is deficient the body will not be able to hold the nutrients which means the food will not be able to stay in the stomach until the digestion process is finalised and the body is no longer able to absorb the nutrients from the food and drink that the person consumes. Hence the person with spleen qi deficiency and spleen yang deficiency will have diarrhoea and loose stool more so than constipation. The diarrhoea could be at any time of the day but will be worse first thing in the morning. The person will need to go to the toilet with urgency when they wake up and the stool will come in a compulsive. This is caused by spleen yang deficiency and also by kidney yang deficiency. Later when I explain about one of the kidney functions of controlling the three orifices, we will discuss this. Night is yin and day is yang and when yang is deficient this means the yang is not able to do its job especially the spleen yang and kidney yang. Generally speaking, spleen yang controls the digestive system and controls what we eat as a food and kidney yang controls the excretion and fluid as a drink. If a person has spleen yang deficiency and kidney yang deficiency they will have, in addition to the diarrhoea and loose stool, puffy swollen eyes with dark circles under the eyelid. Sometimes this condition is caused by lack of sleep. Spleen yang deficiency and kidney yang deficiency can mostly lead to diarrhoea and loose stool but sometimes can also lead to constipation which we will discuss later.

4. Tiredness and exhaustion

The spleen controls our physical strength and also controls our extremities. The muscles need a huge amount of nutrients and fluid to keep our physical strength and energy so that we are able to carry out our daily activities. Our muscular strength comes from the strength of the functional aspect of our spleen which has the job of extracting nutrients and supplying those nutrients to the working muscles and also has the job of extracting the glycogen and glucose which is one of the functions of the liver. If we compare our body to a car our physical energy and physical strength is the car engine, the water in our body represents the water of the car, the oil of the car represents the nutrients our body and the petrol in the car represents the glucose and glycogen which is release by the liver during physical and muscular activity to the working muscles.

5. Bearing down and dragging down sensations

This is when things are collapsing and leads to prolapsed uterus, prolapsed vagina, prolapsed bladder, prolapsed disc, haemorrhoids and heavy vaginal bleeding. All of these are signs that the spleen is not holding in place as it should. One of the functions of the spleen is to keep the organs and tissues in their right place which is the place they are supposed to be in from the first place. This is one of the yang functions of the spleen and also the yang function of the kidney. The spleen has to push the qi and the qi has to push the organs, tissues and blood up to hold them in their correct place. The kidney has to grip the qi and the organs to hold them in their correct place. If a person has spleen yang deficiency the organs and tissues will start to drag down because there is not enough yang to push them up. The function of the yin is to cool and moisten and the function of the yang is to warm and push up which is why all yang channels meet on the top of the head and face.

The yang goes in a vertical direction and the yin goes in a horizontal direction. Yang goes up and yin goes down. If there is spleen yang deficiency and kidney deficiency the organs will start to drag down and descend downwards. This process of dragging and descending downwards of the organs will cause the organs to pass through the weakest point of the tissue.

A slipped disc or hernia are good examples of this scenario. Generally speaking, the disc or hernia will protrude and pass out of the tissue through the weakest point on the body. For example, if you have a weak lower back the disc is more likely to slip out of the lower back than the upper however this also depends on your posture as this will determine the direction that the disc will slip through. If you walk with your neck tilted to the right side it is more likely that the disc in your neck area will slip on the left side and vice versa. The same principal can be applied to the lower back, if you lean or slouch to the right side the disc will slip from the left side. The reason for this is because there is already a physical weakness in the lower back muscles and leaning to the right side will create a further weakness in the muscles and will put huge pressure on the vertebrae and on the disc and because the disc is compressed on the right side it cannot pass through the right side and so starts to move to the left side where it will slip out of its original place.

The same principle applies to any form of hernia. Hernia are defined as the protrusion of the internal tissue through the weaker point in the muscles and the skin. For example, if you have a weakness in your thigh and groin muscles you will have an inguinal hernia which means the tissue protrudes through the thigh and groin muscles. However, if the weakness is in your digestive, respiratory or digestive system these are closer to your chest and diaphragm and means you are more likely to have a hiatus hernia. Belching, burping, heartburn and hiccups over a long period of time might cause hiatus hernia and reflux oesophagitis.

Haemorrhoids are another example of prolapse and occur when the internal tissue of the bowel starts to push out of the back passage. This can happen for two reasons:

•   If a person has constipation and they put a lot of pressure and strain on the bowel when they go to the bathroom for defecation the bowel and the internal tissue will no longer be able to cope with the strain and the pressure and the tissue starts to prolapse out of its original place.

•   Women can often be affected by this condition during pregnancy. One of the functions of the kidneys from an oriental perspective is to control the three orifices, the vagina, the rectum and the penis and also to control pregnancy and labour. The kidney has to grip and hold the qi and the qi has to work hard to push the organ to stay in its correct place. During pregnancy the woman's body is put under a huge amount of pressure both physical and emotional which is caused by so many changes taking place during the pregnancy. One of the physical pressures is caused by the development of the foetus in the womb as the foetus grows it will need more space in the mothers tummy. The heavier the baby becomes the more space that baby will take up and the more dragging and pressure there will be on the mothers tummy and respiratory system. From an oriental perspective the Ren channel is on the front of the body and is yin in nature and descends downwards. The Du channel is on the back of the body and is yang in nature and ascends upwards. The more pressure the Ren channel is out under the harder the Du channel needs to work to keep the organ from descending downward. This explains why the pregnant woman will have a lot of lower back pain and in some severe cases a prolapsed disc also. Pregnant women may also experience frequent urination, diarrhoea or sometimes constipation. Generally speaking, if the woman has more yang deficiency than yin deficiency this will lead to haemorrhoids during pregnancy because as we said earlier the function of the yang is to push and to keep the organs in place. Sometimes the yang deficiency will lead to frequent urination on one hand and to swollen lower limbs and ankle, cellulitis and varicose veins. The disruption of the yang affects the distribution of the body fluid to every channel, organ and tissue down to cellular level therefore if the woman loses a lot of fluid due to frequent urination while pregnant this will be the main reason for her constipation. The fluid is a form of yin and the yin is a form of fluid and both of them have the function to cool and moisten the bowel and when fluid is lost at rapid rate the dryness in the bowel will lead to constipation which in return will lead to haemorrhoids. This could happen at any stage of the pregnancy but especially in the third trimester because in the third trimester the foetus has grown and will descend down to the lower Jiao. The pulse will be slower and the heart rate will be lower and the woman will no longer have morning sickness or vomiting instead she might have frequent urination, constipation, diarrhoea, frequent bowel movements and haemorrhoids which are all part of the pregnancy process. Blood is regarded as an organ from an oriental perspective. The blood should be held in the anterior wall of the veins, arteries and capillaries. Any bleeding which takes place in the body indicates the weakness of the spleen qi whether it is a heavy period, blood or uterine bleeding. If the bleeding is there all the time this means the matter is more serious from a western perspective and there might be a possibility that it is the onset of the cancer in the body regardless of whether the person is male or female. Any form of prolapse whether it is uterus, vagina, bladder or bowel are all linked and connected to the spleen as an organ but mainly it's yang aspect.

6. Chronic bleeding through the bowel movement

7. Heavy period

8. Cold limbs because of spleen yang deficiency

The reason the limbs are cold is because there is not enough spleen qi especially spleen yang qi and kidney yang qi to push the blood around the body's systems and organs hence the body becomes very cold especially the extremities and in particular the legs and feet.

9. Pale tongue and thread weak pulse

The tongue becomes pale because there is not enough spleen qi to push the blood up to the tongue to give it its normal colour which is pink. The pulse becomes thready and is another indication of the weakness of the spleen qi to push the blood and to create the pressure inside the veins, arteries and capillaries.

Cold Damp invading the Spleen

Generally speaking, this is a condition that has the same signs and symptoms of spleen qi deficiency but to a greater extent.

The main causes of this condition are the exposure to the damp cold and to wet. Regardless of whether this cold and damp are coming from the interior or exterior the signs and symptoms are the same. The cold damp invades the body channels and muscles when the person comes into contact with the cold either by sitting on a wet and damp ground or walking in cold water or when the rain invades the body or your clothes get soaking wet. This type of cold attacks and invades the exterior of our body such as the muscles and the channel however there is another type of cold that invades our body and settle sin the interior of our channels and organs. Generally speaking, the interior cold will affect all of our body's systems and organs but from an oriental perspective the main organs affected by interior cold are our kidneys and spleen and will lead to both spleen yang deficiency and kidney yang deficiency. The link between them is the kidney yang deficiency leads to heart yang deficiency and the heart yang deficiency leads to kidney yang deficiency. This means the heart and the kidney will not be harmonised in their physical and functional aspect. The same theory can be applied from a western medicine perspective because if we have a kidney failure, we will have a heart failure and vice versa. The main cause of interior cold apart from the weather is our diet and what we put in our mouth. When you eat raw and cold food or drink anything below room temperature this will undermine our spleen from an oriental perspective and will affect our heart and circulation from an oriental perspective. The treatment method is to warm up the body by tonifying the spleen and the kidney yang and the heart yang and qi. We also ask the client to eat a lot of food that is yang in nature and which will put heat into our system such as chilli, curry, hot spicy food and ginger. We also advise the client to cover their head and ears because most of our body heat leaves the body through the head. Placing a hot water bottle two thumb widths below the bellybutton and another one on the Gate of Vitality on the lower back will help to warm the body. The Gate of Vitality can be found by placing your middle fingers on top of the hips and where your thumbs meet on the back. This is the area where lumbar 4 can be found and where a meningitis test is performed or an epidural injection administered. From an oriental perspective this area represents the kidneys which are basic material for yin and yang. This area is also very rich in nerve endings and blood supply from a western perspective. By warming the belly, you are warming the core and the Ren and by warming the back you are warming the Du, the spine. The Ren channel carries heat to your upper body and the Du channel carries heat to your lower body. The imbalance between these two aspects will create the two extremes between the different channels and organs. From personal experience I see people coming to the clinic with freezing cold hands and the soles of the feet are roasting and vice versa. This could happen at any time and affect any part of the body but will be worse during the winter and in damp winter.

The best way to avoid this condition is to avoid exposure to any cold, wet, damp or windy environment and to be ready and prepared for any climate change.

CHAPTER 9

THE FUNCTION OF THE KIDNEYS

From a western perspective the kidney filters the blood before excretion and the urinary bladder stores and regulates the metabolic rate of body fluid.

The kidneys are a yin organ they work twenty-four hours a day by filtering. They are dense, material and substantial. The paired yang organ to the kidneys is the urinary bladder; it is hollow and is filled and emptied.

From an oriental perspective the kidneys have the following functions:

1. Basic material for yin and yang

2. Produces essence for bone marrow (red blood cells)

3. Controls teeth and nails

4. Water passages (excretion)

5. Controls sexual activity

6. Opens into the three orifices (penis, vagina and rectum)

7. Pregnancy and conception

8. Baby and mother development

9. Opens into the ear (hearing)

10. Gripping the qi

11. Emotion – fear, shock, nervousness and panic

12. Controls courage, willpower, bravery and motivation

13. Manifests in the hair on the head

14. Represents DNA (every kind of DNA)

15. Premature ejaculation

16. Premature greying of hair

1. Basic material for yin and yang

The kidneys are the root of the genetic yin and yang and are the root for every yin and yang aspect in the universe whether it is from an emotional, physical, mental or sexual aspect. The list of yin and yang is endless. You cannot have right without left, up without down, day without night, moon without sun or male without female. Yin and yang are in a constant state of change; they are not static and are interdependent and interchangeable. For example, the transformation of yin to yang and yang to yin can be seen with Ice which is yin, dense and material, when the ice is put into warm water it will melt. The stage of the ice melting is the transformation stage. When the ice is melted it is mixed with the warm water and if you continue to warm the water so it boils the temperature will increase the water will start to evaporate. When the ice was an ice block it was material, substantial and tangible, now the ice and water have evaporated it is non material, non-substantial and non-tangible. This is the transformation of yin to yang. This can be applied to the human body. Anger over a long period of time will lead to the stagnation of qi, one of the liver functions is to ensure the smooth flow of qi, qi pushes blood and blood nourishes qi, if qi is not moving it leads to stagnation and eventually to the formation of a tumour. At the beginning the tumour will be non-malignant but if the person continues to live under pressure and hold onto their emotions regardless of what type of emotion but particularly hatred, resentment, frustration and jealousy which are all related to the liver, the body from an anatomy and physiology perspective will not be able to cope with this emotional state and the bodily functions will diminish. When this happens the cells in the body will refuse to leave the body when their time is up and they become stubborn and this will lead to cancer.

From an oriental perspective every joint in the body is related to an emotion. For example, if you take people who have had knee replacements and you exclude their structural problem and the way they walk most of these people will be stubborn because the knee holds the aspect of being stubborn and is one of the reasons which will contribute to the knee replacement. From an oriental perspective the way how you think will become the way how you feel and the way how you feel will become the way how you think. The way how you think will play a major role in either establishing the tumour in your body or eliminating the tumour out of your body. For example, two people are diagnosed as having non-malignant tumours, one of them is positive and upbeat and cheerful and the other one is negative. Which one is more likely to have the tumour turn cancerous? The answer is the negative person. This is because your negative thoughts will affect all of your bodily functions down to cellular level. The thought is non material, non-substantial and non-tangible which is yang in nature. When everything is gone wrong down to cellular level it will knock all of the bodily functions. There are two types of cells, the red blood cell which carries oxygen and is yin, and the white blood cell which is yang. When you are sick the number of white blood cells increase to fight the infection for you which explains why you look pale when you're sick. The heart has to work harder to c-ordinate with the lymphatic, immune and respiratory systems to defeat the pathogenic invaders. Virus is yin, dormant, no activity and chronic. Bacteria is yang and acute. If we did not have viruses in our body we would die. There are millions of germs and viruses constantly around us. The liver acts like a laser wiping them out before they get to the immune system.

The kidney deals with the urine which is fluid but the function of the kidney is yang because of the movement when it expels the urine and fluid. The yin aspect of the kidney is to cool and moisture and the yang aspect if the kidney is to warm and push. If you have a kidney yin deficiency the cooling and moisture aspect is diminished and this means there is an environment for heat to build up. This heat, whether it is excess or empty, over a long period of time will turn to irritation and inflammation because this environment is suitable for bacteria to grow in. This is why women are more prone to cystitis, kidney infections or bladder infections because of the closeness in location between the vagina and the back passage. Any condition ending in 'it is' means heat and inflammation. No matter what condition the woman comes to you with you need to treat her period. By regulating the woman's period you will improve her health in general.

Progesterone is yang and oestrogen is yin. When a woman is premenstrual the yang will rise. This yang rising is a form of excess and so the woman will have every sign of excess such as headache, irritability and tender breasts. The oestrogen which is yin has the function to cool and moisture and prepares the body for pregnancy and conception. As soon as the period starts al of the symptoms mentioned above will disappear because the progesterone level drops and balance is restored. If the progesterone does not drop and balance is not restored you will continue to have symptoms however this is due to other conditions such as anaemia or psychological conditions.

As I mentioned earlier bleeding is a process of purification and detoxification. When you bleed the first thing the body gets rid of is the toxin, the badness and the stagnation. That explains why from an oriental perspective you have two types of cysts. One is a sac filled with blood and the other is a sac filled with fluid. The cyst filled with blood is more serious and more dangerous that the cyst filled with fluid. This type of cyst filled with blood is more serious and more dangerous that the cyst filled with fluid. This type of cyst along with your emotional state has the potential to turn cancerous. When we talk about the emotional state we mean the way you think and look at things. The cyst filled with fluid does not have the potential to turn cancerous but the bigger it grows it will start to give you discomfort and will begin to push the next organ out of place so that you have prolapse and as we said earlier one of the functions of the spleen is to hold the organs in place and the function of the kidney is to grip the qi and hold it in place.

From an oriental perspective we check the colour of the blood as this can tell us a lot about the condition. If the blood is bright res this is related to deficiency and structural problem such as an injury or sprain. If the blood is dark, black or brown it means there is stagnation in addition to the structural complaint and there is emotional involvement with the condition especially anger. To apply this from a western perspective if you tell your GP that you passed blood in yours tool the GP will ask you the colour of the blood. If the blood is bright red it is coming from external tissue such as haemorrhoids. If the blood is dark or black it is coming from deep inside the body and you might need a colonoscopy or endoscopy to check for something more sinister.

2. Produces essence for bone marrow (Red blood cells)

The essence manufactures blood and regenerates new blood cells. When doctors perform a bone transplant, they take from the femur bone in the thigh and the kidney is related to bones and related to calcium. If your basic constitution that you inherited from your parents is strong then your kidney essence will be strong however if your parent's kidneys essence is weak or your mother is anaemic or didn't eat well throughout the pregnancy then this will affect your kidney essence. The essence represents your constitutional DNA from every aspect whether it is emotional, physical, mental, psychological or sexual. There are two types of essence:

A) Pre Heaven Essence – this essence is inherited from your parents. It is fixed in quality and quantity and you cannot increase it however you can maintain and protect this essence by looking after your health and wellbeing in general such as eating a well-balanced diet, exercising, avoid smoking and alcohol and drinking enough water.

B) Post Heaven Essence – this essence comes from the food you eat and the fluid you drink. It is very important to eat a well-balanced diet to cover all of the five elements which are carbohydrates, protein, fat, vitamins, fluid and minerals. In addition to this it is recommended to avoid eating a lot of red meat. If you don't eat well you may be anaemic and this in turn will affect your post heaven essence and the state of your health and wellbeing in general. It is common to see people with anaemia to also have depression with it.

In women the fluctuation of their hormones during ovulation and menstruation is because progesterone is yang in nature and carbohydrate and sugar are yang in nature also. When a woman is pre-menstrual she will often crave sweet and sugary food because they are trying to create the balance. This is commonly referred to as 'comfort eating' however in reality it is not comfort eating if you did not tackle the root cause of the problem. From an oriental perspective we say the way you think becomes the way you feel and the way you feel becomes the way you think. This means the physical sickness has turned into an emotional sickness even if the physical condition is gone. When dealing with psychological issues you could say that 99% of them are chronic. What I mean by this is, you don't fall asleep one night and wake up the following morning with depression or bipolar disorder or borderline personality disorder etc. Because these issues don't happen overnight.

3. Controls teeth and nails

The teeth are made up of calcium and the nails are made up of keratin and both are related to the kidney function. If you have weak, brittle and thin nails that crack easily this is a sign of three things:

- Kidney qi, essence and yin deficiency
- Blood and essence deficiency
- Deficiency of vitamins and minerals

A weakness in kidney essence and kidney qi will lead to:

- Delay in baby teeth coming in
- Weak teeth that fall out easily
- Premature dental fillings

The condition may be hereditary if, for example, the mother has osteoporosis because then the baby may be born with weak teeth and bones. The teeth are considered an extension of the bones.

Diet is another factor that may affect the condition. The more fizzy and sweet drinks you consume the faster you will destroy your teeth. Also eating a lot of red meat, drinking a lot of alcohol and smoking will destroy your teeth.

4. Water passages (Excretion)

The kidneys regulate the water passages through the process of excretion of body fluids. The kidney is a yin organ and its paired yang organ is the urinary bladder. The urinary bladder stores urine and the kidneys expel urine. The more water you drink the more the kidneys have to expel. From an oriental perspective it is not good if your urine is pale and colourless and you are not drinking water because this means that your body is not holding the nutrients. One of the functions of the kidneys is to regulate calcium, potassium, magnesium, and sodium and all of these will be lost during the process. If your urine is yellow and has a strong smell and you are drinking water this means there is a lot of protein and bacteria in the urine which after a long period of time may lead to a kidney or bladder infection.

Generally speaking if the urine is pale and colourless this means there is a kidney yang deficiency and if the urine is yellow and strong smelling this means there is heat whether excess or empty heat. The kidneys have a huge link with every organ particularly the heart. From an oriental perspective there is a condition called 'Kidney and Heart not harmonised'. The same can be said to apply from a western perspective because kidney failure is accompanied by heart failure and heart failure will be accompanied by kidney failure. This is because the kidney filters the toxins from the blood before it is sent to the heart so that the heart won't be circulating toxins, such as the build-up of protein and acid, around the body.

5. Sexual activity

The kidneys control the sexual activity and the sexual desire from both the male and female perspective. Sexual activity from an oriental perspective is not only related to the reproductive system. The reproductive system is like a mirror that reflects your emotional state and the state of your health and wellbeing in general but especially the state of your sexual activity and sexual organs. The person will have cold hands and feet, frequent urination, weak lower back, lack of sexual desire, lack of affection and pre-mature ejaculation. If the person has heat, whether excess or empty heat, and the heat has invaded the kidneys as an organ and the reproductive as a system the person will have slight sweating especially from the soles of the feet and sometimes from the palms of the hands, yellow smelly urine, tinnitus, weakness of hearing, excessive sexual desire with no satisfaction or contentment, they will either not be able to climax or will have sexual activity and will crave more and more with no satisfaction or fulfilment. Sometimes from an oriental perspective this is not related to anything physical because physically both people may be perfect but they don't have any emotional compatibility between them. As we said earlier, you cannot force anybody to have feelings for you. Why? Because you could make one hundred people wake up from sleeping but you can't make one-person sleep because that is up to them. That explains why some people with insomnia and who use insomnia tablets end up committing suicide. You can't make somebody love you but you can make somebody hate you. Love is yin and gradual, and hatred is yang and acute. Hatred is up to you and love belongs to them and vice versa. For example, if you take a needle and you poke somebody with it they will get angry, you have been able to make them angry or upset at you in a matter of seconds, however you could not make them love you in a matter of seconds.

From an oriental perspective it is completely opposite to the western perspective when they say 'we make love'. From an oriental perspective this does not make any sense because love and sexual activity are completely two separate things. You might have sexual activity with someone you don't love and you might not have sexual activity with someone you do love. Of course it will make a difference when you have sexual activity with someone you have feelings for and they have feelings for you. Lack of sexual desire, excessive sexual desire, premature ejaculation and impotence are all related and linked to the kidneys from an oriental perspective.

6. Opens into the three orifices

The kidneys open into the three orifices which are the penis, vagina and rectum. One of the functions of the kidneys is to grip the qi. If kidney qi is weak the orifices will not be able to open and close at the right time and so might open at the wrong time and close at the wrong time. This is equivalent to the sphincter muscle from a western perspective which is responsible for opening and closing when you pass urine or when you have bowel movement. Weak kidney qi along with kidney yang deficiency will lead to heavy periods in a woman. The orifices are wide open and they are not able to close up at the right time and this is why sometimes the woman will have excessive urination and diarrhoea with their period. At other times when the woman is pre-menstrual, she may have scanty urination. This will depend on the kidney qi and kidney yang when the period starts. From a western perspective it depends on the progesterone and oestrogen level. Progesterone is yang and responsible for starting the period, oestrogen is yin and is responsible for starting pregnancy and preparing the lining of the womb.

7. Pregnancy and conception

Pregnancy and conception depend on the three aspects of the kidneys which are qi, yin and yang but especially on kidney qi. The kidneys are located in the lower back on the Du channel and the urinary bladder is located on the front of the body and on the Ren channel. These locations explain why a woman needs the following for a healthy labour:

➤ Strong spine, especially the lower back
➤ Strong core
➤ Strong lungs
➤ Strong circulation
➤ Strong emotional state and state of mind

If a woman has weakness in her back and stomach this is one of the reasons that can lead to miscarriage. The body is either physically not able to start the pregnancy or the woman is able to get pregnant but she is not able to maintain the pregnancy, the woman might have a number of miscarriages in a short period of time and the stage of the miscarriage will determine the constitutional weakness of the kidneys as an organ and the lower back and the core. The longer the woman holds the baby before the miscarriage occurs the more emotional attachment she will have with the baby and the more of an impact the miscarriage will have on her. Of course, both parents will feel disappointed and have a sense of sadness and grief but the parent who takes longer to recover will be worse in the long run.

Posture is very important to achieve a healthy pregnancy and that is why we advise a lot of women to do yoga classes during pregnancy. The yoga practitioner will give them specific exercises depending on the stage of their pregnancy. The state of woman's mind and her emotional feelings will also determine the state and health of the new-born baby.

8. Opens into the ear

The kidneys open into the ears and control our sense of hearing. The kidneys are related to our DNA which is our genetic material that we inherit from our parents. The first sense established as a baby is the sight and the last sense established is the hearing. This is while the baby is still in the womb. When we are born and when we get older the cycle will reverse, the first sense that we lose is our sight and the last sense we lose is our hearing. The stronger your kidney essence, qi, yin and yang are, the stronger your hearing will be.

If one of your kidneys is removed, regardless of the reason why, in some cases this will affect your hearing in general but especially the opposite ear to the kidney removed. For example, if you have your left kidney removed then your hearing in your right ear might be affected and vice versa.

Sometimes hearing problems can be due to deformities or they can be hereditary which means it might run in the family and this goes back to the persons structural and physical DNA which is related to our kidneys as an organ from an oriental perspective.

9. Gripping the Qi

The lungs descend qi, the kidneys grip qi, the liver moves the qi in a wave and the spleen has to move the qi upwards from the toes to the head which is equivalent to the heart from a western perspective. From an oriental perspective there are two types of asthma, yin asthma and yang asthma. If you are not able to breathe out this type of asthma is related to the lungs and to sadness and grief and is related to weakness of lung qi which leads to weakness of the lung function and in return this will affect your exhalation process. The other type of asthma is related to the kidneys. If you are having difficulty breathing in it means the kidneys are not gripping the qi and is related to shock and fear. Kidney qi deficiency will lead to weakness in all of the spine especially in the lower back and also weakness of the three orifices. When the orifices are weakened their functions will be affected. There is an exercise which can be done to strengthen the yin and the yang. The Du channel is a yang channel and is related to the kidneys and the spine on the back of the body, the Ren channel is a yin channel and is related to the urinary bladder, core and front of the body. All of the extremities also have to be strengthened especially the lower limbs. The exercise to do this is similar to pretend cycling and can be done lying on your back on the floor. When you bring your leg up into the air you are pushing the circulation back from the toes to the heart, this represents the venous return of the blood and is against the direction of gravity. As we mentioned earlier if a woman wears shoes with high heels this will make her back weaker and it will be more difficult for the circulation to go back up.

10. Emotion – fear, shock, panic

The kidneys are related to shock, fear and panic and to any state of being afraid or nervous. A good example of this is when you have a job interview and you feel nervous and you start to run to the toilet to urinate. If we take you to the laboratory to examine your kidneys and bladder, structurally from an anatomy and physiology perspective there will be nothing wrong with them. The question is from an oriental perspective what makes you urinate a lot? The answer is because the kidneys are related to fear and the fear has an emotional effect on the kidney function which makes you have frequent urination. The same applies from a western perspective when we talk about adrenalin. There are two glands on top of the kidneys called the adrenal glands which produce adrenalin to balance the homeostasis, this means to balance the external environment with the internal environment. For example, if a person is afraid of dogs they will become afraid and panic when they see a dog running towards them. The dog is the external provoking factor to the internal state of the body. When the dog is gone and the cause of the fear is no longer there the body will go back to its own original state. However sometimes even when the body goes back to its original state the shock is trapped in the body and the organs will pay the price for it especially the kidney, heart and lungs. This is why sometimes when people hear happy news, they will drop dead with a heart attack and also when people hear sad news they also drop dead with a heart attack. This is the mutual consumption of them at the same time when the person heard the news.

The kidneys open into the three orifices and also controls the conception and labour. If one woman falls pregnant as a result of rape and another woman falls pregnant with a loving partner, from an anatomy and physiology perspective both of them will have to pass through exactly the same process, conception, labour, delivery and baby. The difference between these two women is that shock as an emotion will play a major part in all of the process from the beginning to the end and in return will play a major part in the mothers health and in the health of the new born baby.

11. Kidneys control Courage, Willpower and Motivation

The kidneys as an organ control courage, willpower and motivation. As we said earlier, when a woman has a miscarriage it is related to a weakness in her kidneys and spleen energies, especially kidney yang and spleen energies. The motivation is related to the kidneys because sometimes you have energy but you have no motivation and vice versa. For example, you might have the energy to buy the newspaper but you do not have the motivation to read it. This means your spleen energy is predominant because the spleen controls the physical energy. Sometime you might have the motivation but you don't have the physical energy to do it, for example to walk. This means the kidney is over predominant on the spleen. The best example can be seen in people with ME (chronic fatigue syndrome), sometimes they have the motivation to go for a walk but they don't have the physical energy. If their condition gets too bad they will not have the energy or the motivation. The motivation will support your willpower and vice versa. The willpower is the will to do something or to achieve something. This is applied to everything from emotional, physical and mental. This also applies to people who are terminally ill. In the case of terminally ill people if their kidney qi is strong and their will power and motivation is strong they will be able to overcome it. In the case of terminally ill people if their kidney qi is strong and their willpower and motivation is strong, they will be able to overcome their chronic terminal condition. It is completely opposite for the terminally ill people who reach a stage and they will lose their will to live, this is why they lose their will to live and they will not be interest in doing anything or trying anything. Courage and willpower are opposite to fear and to having no willpower. For example, as we said earlier, the courage and the will power could be established by the way you are brought up by your parents. If your parents have a fear of everything this will pass onto their children. A child establishes their own identity as a unique human and they could overcome this by doing the opposite to what they were told not to do. For example, if a child is told not to swim because it is dangerous, now the child as an adult has a decision to make and the determination, motivation and willpower will support their decision to have the courage to go on and learn how to swim. The reason I am saying this is so that they do not pass it on their own children. Generally speaking, the emotional and psychological problems are problems that are not inherited, they are not hereditary. If a person's father has fear this does not mean that the person themselves also have fear, it will not be a part of their physical makeup or physical DNA. However, if a woman has a shock during pregnancy this shock could affect the new-born baby but if she is pregnancy with twins it might only affect one baby. We do not know why this is because we do not have the answer for everything. All we know is that from personal experience we see people who have a twin or triplets and one of them will be very brace and outgoing and outspoken and the other is completely the opposite, shy, nervous and introverted. All of these psychological and emotional conditions are related back to our kidneys because the kidneys represent our DNA.

12. Opens into the hair of the head

The hair and the nails are an extension of the kidneys and they represent the kidney qi. The hair of the body is related to the lungs and the hair of the head is related to the kidneys. The kidneys represent our DNA which is the constitutional material that we inherit from our parents. This explains why if a person has chemotherapy or radiation therapy in some cases the hair of the head falls out and sometimes all the hair on the body. This will depend on what type of cancer the person has and how aggressive it and also what stage the cancer is at because there are four stages of cancer. Chemotherapy and radiation therapy demolish the DNA and because the hair represents the DNA the hair starts to fall out. Because the DNA demolished, we have to start all over again like a new-born baby. The stronger the hair is the stronger the kidney qi, yin, yang and essence is and vice versa.

If your hair falls out easily when you comb it means there is an imbalance in the hormonal system from a western perspective. If the hair is dry this is related to blood deficiency, yin deficiency and yang deficiency and sometimes to the pre essence from an oriental perspective. The pre heaven essence will influence and affect the hair on the head and this is why some people from the same families will have the same kind of hair. From a female aspect if the hair falls out easily when it is combed it means that there is a lack of vitamins along with a hormonal imbalance, and it can also be related to the menstrual cycle. The heavier the woman's period is and the more blood that is lost will result in weaker hair and it will affect the quantity and quality of her hair.

13. Represents DNA

The kidneys represent the DNA which is the genetic material we inherit from our parents. From an oriental perspective we do not talk about DNA from an anatomy and physiology perspective, instead we talk about the emotional and physical DNA that you inherit from your parents. During pregnancy the woman will pass every sort of emotion through the umbilical cord to the baby. The reason for all the emotions is due to the fluctuation of the woman's hormones and the fluctuation of her emotional state and the state of her feeling in general. For example, the lungs are related to sadness and grief and they control the skin, if the mother has sadness and grief during the pregnancy, she will pass her emotional DNA onto the baby. If the mother is tall and blonde this might be the physical DNA, she will pass to the baby along with the father's DNA. This explains why some babies have eczema or psoriasis from the first day they are born and at the same time they have asthma.

This is because the two emotions, sadness and grief, are hugely linked to the respiratory as a system and to the lungs and skin as organs. If the mother has a lot of excitement and happiness this will affect the new-born baby's heart because the heart from an oriental perspective is related to happiness and excitement. This explains why sometimes when people hear happy news their heart will start to beat faster. As we said, the lungs are related to sadness and grief and the heart is related to happiness and excitement, both the heart and lungs are located in the upper Jiao portion of the body. Some people will hear sad news, they will drop dead with a heart attack, some people hear happy news and they drop dead with a heart attack, from an oriental perspective this represents the mutual consumption of the yin and the yang at the same time the person heard the news. By this I mean the mutual consumption of the yin and the yang of the same organ because the heart has yang and also yin and the lungs also have yin and yang. The imbalance between two forces, the yin and the yang, will lead to the outcome and the consequences. Oriental medicine is all about balancing the yin and the yang from every aspect whether emotional, physical or mental to achieve the optimum level of health and wellbeing.

14. Pre-mature greying

Pre-mature greying of the hair is related to a weakness in kidney qi and kidney essence. There will also be contributing factors such as your lifestyle, the way you eat, what you eat, whether you smoke or drink, the amount of exercise you do and the type of life you live in general. If life is very stressful and if you don't get enough sleep it will contribute to the pre-mature greying of hair. However sometimes grey hair is inherited from your parents and therefore can be hereditary.

15. Pre-mature ejaculation

Weakness in kidney qi especially kidney yang qi will lead to either impotence or pre-mature ejaculation. This is related to a weakness of kidney qi and to the weakness of the spine, stomach and circulation in general. This explains why people who expose themselves to a very cold and damp environment will have their kidneys affected whether it is the yin or the yang aspect. In return this will lead to weakness in all the reproductive system and this will lead to pre-mature ejaculation. As we now know the kidneys are related to shock and sometimes shock will also affect the reproductive system in general resulting in the man not being able to get an erection in the first place or he might have pre-mature ejaculation. There are also other causative factors such as being shy or nervous or inexperienced in all of your life in general including your sexual life.

The Kidneys from a five-element perspective
Direction – North

The kidneys represent the direction of north and they also represent the cold. The opposite of the kidneys is the heart which represents the south and heat. the kidney channel starts on the sole of the feet and ends below the heart. If you sit in a damp and cold place you will have yang deficiency symptoms such as weak back, poor memory, no headaches, premature ejaculation, cold extremities and frequent urination. If you have kidney yin deficiency there will be nothing to cool and moisture and you will have cystitis, kidney infections, bladder infections and kidney stones. From an oriental perspective the kidneys represent the lymphatic, immune and endocrine system.

The kidneys are related to the cold and to winter. People feel depressed in the winter because the vitamin D from the sun is not there. This is why people go on holidays and it makes them feel better. The amount of vitamin A you get depends on your skin type. If you are very fair skinned and you have too much exposure to the sun this can lead to skin cancer. It is very rare to find a black person getting skin cancer and if they do it will not serious. Winter will affect your emotional state and the state of your mind. Your mind will begin to wander and when it does it will have no limitations. The mind does not know the different between right and wrong. If the mind knows that anxiety is of no good it does not know how to deal with it. This is because the mind is space less, weightless, timeless and limitless and every minute it has thousands of ideas and thoughts to process.

Any imbalance in the magnesium, sodium, potassium and calcium which the kidneys have to regulate will affect all of your health in general including your mind. For example, too much salt leads to high blood pressure, not enough salt leads to low blood pressure. Too much calcium leads to an irregular heart beat and subsequently a heart attack, not enough calcium leads to osteoporosis. Potassium and magnesium affect our body functions deep down to cellular level and affect the electrolytes of the cells.

Taste – Salt

The kidneys control the salty taste. Excess heat in the kidneys will lead to excessive craving for salt with frequent urination. In this case you are eating a lot of salt but your body is not holding it. This means there is weakness in the kidneys. The kidneys have to regulate the metabolic rate of body fluid, meaning excretion.

Too much salt will mean the kidneys are under a lot of pressure and this will result in scanty urine, cystitis, constipation and scanty periods. Where there is not enough salt it is the opposite, low blood pressure, pale and colourless urine and frequent urination.

The kidneys control the calcium, magnesium, potassium and sodium. If we have a kidney failure, we will also have a heart failure. The heart controls sweating, when we exercise, we sweat a lot and an imbalance between the kidneys in excretion and the heart in circulating may occur. When you sweat you lose fluid and sodium and you might get cramps and spasms. This because the calcium, magnesium, potassium and sodium are needed for the muscular contraction. Too much salt being lost will lead to an imbalance which goes down to cellular level and will affect how the muscles work. The muscles work in pairs and not as individuals. An example of this is the biceps and triceps in the upper arms. When the biceps relax the triceps have to contract and vice versa. When there is not enough salt and fluid there will be cramps, spasms and stiffness. The muscles will contract and it will not be able to relax. The question from an oriental perspective is why does the muscle contract (go into spasm) and not relax? The answer is because the kidneys are the basic nutrient material for the yin and the yang and this goes all the way down to cellular level including nutrient level. Calcium is yin and potassium is yang. If you only eat dairy products you will have dampness, headaches, mucus, migraine and vertigo. If you eat only bananas which are potassium and no dairy products you will have constipation because the kidneys will be under pressure dealing with the potassium.

It is good to sweat however there are three types of sweating:

1) Sweating while doing cardiovascular exercise. This is the co-ordination between the kidneys as an organ and the skin as an organ.

2) Sweating with no physical activity. This means there is weakness in the heart and disharmony between the heart and the kidney.

3) Sweating when you go a sauna. This is not good if you already have low blood pressure because you will lose salt when you sweat and it could lead to a heart attack. However, it can be good for you if you have high blood pressure because you have excess salt.

Colour – Black and Grey

In wintertime the day is shorter and this means the sunsets earlier and the night hours will be longer than the day time hours and the colour will be black and grey. The kidney is related to the moon, north and cold and the heart is related to the south and to heat. In winter time you will find that you urinate more often. This is because in the summer you lose fluid through the sweating process through the skin so there is not much fluid to be extracted through urination.

Winter time as a season with dark as the colour and grey cloud as the environment will affect our mood and the state of our health and wellbeing. It will even affect our thoughts and the way we see and look at things. This is because of the lack of vitamin D from the sun which will affect our perception and the perception will influence our projection whether from a western perspective or from an oriental perspective.

Age – Old

As we said earlier the liver is related to spring and presents the new born baby, the heart represents the summer and the youth, the lungs represent metal and the stage of growing up and the kidneys represent winter and the old age. The baby stage is the first stage in life and the old age is the last stage in life before death. Our body is not designed to live forever or for this life. Our body is designed to live for a certain number of years. You could influence your age by your lifestyle, anything you do with your lifestyle will affect your body and your age in general. Certain organs pay the price for certain problems, for example smoking will damage your body in general but especially the liver, eating hot and spicy food and pork will affect your stomach. Another example is using a lot of makeup on your face which will speed up the ageing process because when you put chemicals and makeup on your skin you are not allowing the skin to receive enough oxygen.

From an oriental perspective the ageing process can be compared to a set of CD's (compact discs). If you have one hundred CDs and each CD represents a year in your life then the first cd represents the core and the centre of the cell, the nucleus and nucleolus. If you copy the cd then more the quality of the cd will deteriorate because you are moving away from the core, nucleus and nucleolus of the cell. For example, if you ran when you are twenty and you run again when youare forty your arteries at forty are narrower and the heart has to pump harder. Your ligaments, cartilageand tendons will also have lost their elasticity and flexibility and the joint will be affected. The old age is the stage where the wheel turns back again. You are born with no teeth and now at this stage the teeth will fall out. When you were a baby you were not able to walk, now in old age it is the same and you might needto go back to thestage where you needed to crawl. In a baby the memory is being established, in old age the memory is declining especially the short term memory which is related to your spleen. A baby is born with no hair and when we get old the hair starts to fall out. A baby's sight is weak and the muscles tries to get stronger by focusing on objects they look at, similarly when you get older the sight begins to go the same way. The last sense established in the human body is the hearing and the last sense we lose when we are elderly is the hearing.

After the old age is the stage of death the spleen and the stomach represent the earth, at the stage of death they are gone back to the grave, the way that they started.

To recap:

The liver is wood and wood goes into the fire. The heart is fire. When the wood is burned it turns into metal. The lungs are metal and the metal turns to water. Water is store in the kidneys. Water goes back again into the ground. This is the circle of life, from yin to yang and from yang to yin, from youth to old and old to youth and from life to death and death to life. You are born when you die and you die when you are born.

Sound – Groaning

This is the state of being pessimistic and unhappy. It is similar to being in a state of depression because of the chemical and hormonal imbalance. This is opposite to the stats where you are excited and your voice is loud and you are cheerful and upbeat. Generally speaking everything could be rectified by looking after the body from every aspect whether it is emotional, physical, mental or sexual and looking after our health and well-being in general. It all goes back to balancing the yin with the yang and that is what oriental medicine is all about.

The end of the book. Thank God endlessly as every second is a gift from God the Creator.

FROM PREVIOUS BOOKS

HUMAN REPLICATION

From an anatomy physiology perspective, every finger represents a toe; the thumb represents the big toe, the index finger represents the second toe, the middle finger represents the middle toe, the ring finger represents the fourth toe, and the little finger represents the little toe. The palm of the hand represents the sole of the foot; the back of the hand represents the back of the foot; the wrist represents the ankle, the radius bone (arm) represents the tibia (leg), and the ulna (arm) represents the fibula (leg); the elbow represents the knee; the biceps and triceps (arm muscles) represent the thigh and quads (leg muscles). The shoulders represent the hip. In regards to the head, each side of the brain, is connected to the gluteus; the left side of the brain controls the right side of the body, and vice-versa. We have 32 teeth, and 32 ribs, every tooth represents a rib. The lips represent the reproductive system, especially the vagina; the tongue represents the penis. The viscera (internal organs) come together as Yin and Yang.

On the back the urinary bladder channel is the biggest channel on the human body: starting from the inside corner of the eye it goes all the way up to the top of the head, circulates twice around the spine, and goes all the way down to the small toe. One and a half thumbs beside the spine, are the physical points which are connected to the organs and the nerves that they are linked to.

Points that are three thumb measures beside the spine are emotional and psychological points; these points are related to the way we feel, think, act and behave.

As mentioned earlier, from an Oriental perspective, every organ represents an emotion, and it controls the tissue connected to this emotion. Sometimes when I lecture about human replication I get asked this question: *"You say the gallbladder is related to decision-making, and the kidneys are related to fear. Does this mean, if a person's gallbladder is surgically removed, they continue making the wrong decisions for the rest of the life?"*

The answer is *'no'*, for the following reasons:

1. When we talk about the gallbladder from an Oriental perspective, we are not only talking from an anatomical and physiological perspective or from a physical point of view. We are also looking at the emotional aspect, the aspect related to human feelings.

2. If the gallbladder is surgically removed, regardless of the reason, whether it is due to damage, a tumour, or gallstones, etc., the gallbladder meridian remains and will take over the organ aspect. The same applies to the kidneys, which are related to fear, panic and any form of phobia. Somebody from a medical background asked me the same question, about the kidneys this time, he said to me, "if you say that the kidneys represent courage from an oriental perspective, does this mean the person will be a coward for the rest of his life, because his kidneys have been removed, regardless of the reason?" Also, the answer is 'no', because we don't talk about the kidneys from a structural point of

view, we talk about the emotional aspect which is connected to the kidneys as an organ, and in addition the person still has the kidney channel which will take over the process.

In Oriental medicine, there are a variety of ways to diagnose. One of the strongest tools of diagnosis are the tongue and the pulse diagnosis. However, sometimes people come to the clinic and either have no arms, and we cannot check the pulse in their arm; or they are paralysed and there is no feeling or sensation when we put our hand on their wrist to check for their pulse. In this case, the lower limbs will take over. From a structural and emotional aspect, also, that explains why you see some people whose arms are paralysed start writing with their feet, using a pen. The other way of diagnosis is tongue diagnosis. There are people who come to the clinic, who either can't stick their tongue out, or have a face injury which makes it impossible for them to open their mouth in the first place. In this case, the energy from the tongue is transferred to the channel representing the tongue, which is the heart and pericardium channel. The energy is transferred and with it the emotional aspect and the emotional feeling. We are not talking about the structural aspect of the tongue, as a muscle. Another question that I get asked is, *'How do you prove, from an Oriental perspective, that every area of the tongue represents an internal organ from a physical point of view, and represents the emotional state which is linked to this organ from an oriental point of view?'*

Please read the following very carefully:

1. One of the heart functions, from an oriental perspective and from a five-element point of view, is that it opens into the tongue, and controls the tongue. The heart circulates blood to every organ and to every part of the human body, from the top of

the head to the sole of the feet. The heart also captures the mind, which is the non-physical aspect of the brain and represents our state of mind and the state of our emotional feeling. The heart circulates blood. The blood carries our state of mind to every part of our body, down to cellular level. That explains why the structural, functional and emotional state of all our internal organs, and consequently the state of our general health and wellbeing, is reflected on our tongue. This is the link from an oriental perspective.

2.   That explains why, from an Oriental perspective, we have two types of heart attack: The Yin and the Yang heart attack. When the tongue drops to the left, it is a Yang heart attack, and when the tongue drops to the right, it is a Yin heart attack. The heart controls the movements of the tongue; this means it oversees our speech. When we talk about speech, we don't mean general talk. We mean the total clarity of our pronunciation which makes it easy for other people to understand us. Hence, when the person has a heart attack, their speech may be slurred. Also, because the heart captures the mind, and the mind will be disturbed, the person will be disoriented. From a Western perspective, this is the case not only because the heart attack occurred, but also because the heart attack deprived the brain of oxygen.

3.   The tongue is a muscle in the human body that can do any movement and in any direction.

4.   Every other muscle in our body has two points: the point of origin, and the point of insertion. For example, the biceps muscle – this also applies to all the other muscles in our body because they work in the same way. The point of origin is the point where the muscle touches the bone, and does not move. In

regards to the biceps, the point of origin is the head of the humerus (the top of the upper arm), and the point of insertion is the point where the muscle is attached to the tendon and moves the next joint and whatever is attached to it. In the case of the biceps, the point of insertion is the ulna. That explains why your arm straightens up when you move your biceps. The tongue is the only exception in the human body. Why is that? Because the tongue does not have a point of insertion, it only has a point of origin, which is attached to our upper jaw.

5. The tongue has millions of nerve endings, which are connected to all our senses, e.g. the sense of taste. Gastric enzymes are produced in the mouth, with the help of the tongue, saliva and teeth (through the chewing process) they aid the digestion process. The longer food is being chewed in the mouth, the less work the stomach must do. The tongue is a huge link to our sense of smell. To prove this, I will give you this very simple example: the appetite of people who smoke is affected by the smoking and their sense of smell is either decreased or gone completely. In turn, this affects their taste as a sense and their digestive system in general but especially the stomach and the lungs. Because when the person smokes, the lungs are affected by the carbon dioxide, which is produced through the smoking process, and causes the lungs to become dry. As far as we know, the lungs should be moist. The cavity surrounding the lungs is called the pleura, which carries fluid to help with the breathing process and to prevent friction. Dryness in the lungs in turn will cause dryness in the stomach, because the lungs must take oxygen and pump it to the heart, and the heart must circulate oxygen to all organs. The next organ which comes immediately after the heart is the stomach. When the blood is filled with

carbon dioxide, which is caused by the inhalation of smoke, this carbon dioxide will travel to all body parts, but especially to the stomach. This will lead to dryness and ulcers, indigestion, belching, burping, hiccups, and in turn the person's appetite will be affected. That explains why, people's appetite increases after they stop smoking. They start to eat more and put on weight, because their sense of taste and sense of smell is linked to the tongue through the heart, their circulation will also improve a lot. This is the reason why people are sometimes afraid to stop smoking: the fear of putting on weight. We tell these people that, from an oriental perspective, we have a specific point we can use to decrease or suppress their appetite. We have a lot of people who come to the clinic to lose weight, some of these people lost five or six stones, only by receiving acupuncture treatments, following the instructions we give them, and breathing the new way of breathing that we teach them.

People ask, how does this work? The answer is because all our actions are done by the brain. How e.g. do we feel hungry? The message goes from the brain to the stomach, and you start to eat. When you are full, the message must go back from the stomach to the brain to tell you to stop eating. When we use a specific point, we access the subconscious mind and we go to the root cause, which makes the person eat in the first place. That explains why people tell you 'I lost three stones when I joined the gym, but as soon as I stopped, I start to put the weight back on again.' From an oriental perspective, this is not the case. After the initial consultation with the person, and after checking their tongue and pulse, which are some of the most important tools in diagnosing a condition from an oriental perspective, we find out the root cause that initiated the person's eating habit. We use specific acupuncture points, which are mostly psychological and emotional points. These put the brain in charge of all processes, down to the subconscious level and down to a deep emotion cellular level. When we use these points, the brain will decide how many calories the person who wants to lose weight needs per their physical activity. E.g., a builder needs to go up and down the stairs 100 times during the day. His brain will decide what his body needs, depending on his physical activity. In comparison to this a woman who is sitting in the office answering the phone all day, will not need the same number of calories that the builder needs, the brain will decide.

How do we prove this from an Oriental perspective? When we link it to the human body, from an anatomy physiology point of view, and from a western medical perspective, we talk about the endocrine system and hormones, especially the thyroxin hormone, which represents the Yang aspect from an oriental perspective, and the metabolic rate from a western perspective. This explains why, from an oriental perspective, there are people who eat very little, but they still put on a lot of weight, especially those who have an underactive thyroid. These people feel bloated, their body is very puffy, especially under their eyes, their ankles might be swollen, and their circulation might be affected. Most of the time, they have weakness in their kidneys, which leads to an imbalance, and they either must urinate very often, or they suffer from fluid retention all over their body, especially on their extremities but mainly their legs. They always feel cold, especially their feet. Completely opposite to this is the person who has an overactive thyroid. This person has Yin deficiency which leads to too much heat in the body down to cellular level. This heat leads to hyperactivity, which explains why in most cases the person has a very fast heart rate and pulse. They feel hot, and their skin looks red, especially their face and cheeks. People with an underactive thyroid have Yang deficiency, that means they have cold in their body. That explains why they feel cold most of the time, and they have a very white, pale complexion. This is the link from an oriental perspective: the heart opens into the tongue, and the heart controls the circulation and the complexion in general, especially of the face. This matches your saying: 'cold hands, warm heart'. This means in your own way; you are talking about the heart and circulation. As I mentioned earlier, the right side of the body is controlled by the left side of the brain, and vice-versa. This means the muscular movements and the joint movements on the right side of the body are controlled by the left side of the brain, and vice-versa. The only exception is the tongue, because the tongue is the only muscle that does not belong to either side. The tongue controls all our senses. All our senses are controlled by and connected to the tongue. As I mentioned earlier, the people who smoke, their sense of smell and taste is affected by the smoking which in turn affects their digestive system and their stomach as an organ, and their appetite in general. That explains why some people are afraid to quit smoking, because they are afraid of putting on weight. This means there is a psychological fear of solving one problem because it might create another one. All of us could have this kind of psychological fear no matter if we are smokers or not. From an oriental perspective, we ask this question: Why do some people eat like a horse, and do not put on any weight and other people eat very little, but put on weight. From an Oriental perspective, this leads to the following conclusion: not everybody who is overweight or obese eats a lot. This means there may be a psychological reason behind putting on the weight. This psychological reason will represent the psychological Yin of obesity and the psychological Yang of obesity. The psychological Yin of obesity represents the type of people who eat without being hungry and for psychological reasons. Some people eat when they are angry, others when they are sad, others when they are bored, this is called 'comfort eating', but in fact it is 'discomfort eating'. We call it a discomfort eating because the food does not heal or fix their psychological problems which are deeply imbedded within them, down to cellular level; as some people say 'Your issue is in your tissue'. What I mean by this is people who say they eat because they are angry, still have their anger after eating. The same applies to sadness, boredom, and the list is endless. What is most interesting from an oriental perspective, when we backtrack the habit of 'comfort' eating, it goes back to the day we were born, even further back, to the days before we were born. Remember when I was talking about how the mother's emotional state and emotional feeling, her lifestyle and her habits are passed on to her new-born baby through the umbilical cord and will be part of the baby, regardless of gender? A simple example therefore is: you might find out that the baby likes sweets because the mother likes sweets and craved and ate them during her pregnancy. The same applies to foods she did not like. Hence, these two eating habits will already be established and ready made for the new baby to start their life with. But either way, people could be helped with unhealthy eating habits by changing and breaking their habit. Sometimes the habit of overeating is related to the way you were brought up and your parents' lifestyle. What I mean by this is the following: Sometimes when the baby cries, the parents choose the easiest option by giving the baby food to eat to stop them from crying, without finding the root cause of their crying. The same applies when babies are given the soother a lot. This can backfire in some cases, because it provides them with a false feeling of being fed. This might initiate the habit of excess eating in the future, which can result in gaining excess weight. To prove this in a very simple and easy way I will give you the following example: if the baby was crying because s/he was sad or upset, and was given food to eat, later in life the baby will associate the feeling of being upset and sad with the habit of indulging in any kind of food, which can result in becoming overweight or obese. In their mind, they think it is comfort eating. Same applies to any other emotion which makes the baby cry, regardless of the reason. For example, associating the anger state with the eating habit, the emotional list is endless.

NOTES

DHEAI'S ESSENTIALS

THE BREATH OF FIRE

The aim of 'the breath of fire' is to create the balance between breathing in and breathing out. This strengthens the function of the respiratory, circulatory and lymphatic system. It helps the lungs function to their optimum level when extracting oxygen and expelling carbon dioxide, which in turn improves our general health and wellbeing, including medical conditions that people present themselves to the clinic with. That explains why every medical condition gets worse if we breath fast and improves if we breath slowly. Most of us have no problem breathing in but our problem is breathing out properly. No matter how shallow or weak our breathing is, we still take in oxygen. The problem however starts when we are unable to expel the carbon dioxide that builds up inside our body. Per the Middle Eastern philosophy and from an emotional perspective breathing out holds the aspect of letting go, regardless of what emotion or feeling we are holding onto.

HOW IT IS DONE:

The breath of fire is a short fast sniffing breath; moving the lungs, the ribs and the diaphragm in a pumping movement while inhaling and exhaling the air forcefully through the nose.

After mastering the breath of fire, you can use your thumb and index finger to pinch your nose and open and close your nostrils, allowing the air to pass in and out of the nose. This helps open your sinuses, which are the first gate in your respiratory system, supporting your lungs and respiratory system to function to their optimum level and hence improving your health and wellbeing in general.

POSTURE

Be careful of your posture, while lying, sitting, standing or walking. The spine is considered the body's scaffolding. Bad posture worsens any kind of medical condition, whilst good posture helps improve ailments and medical conditions.

GENERAL TIPS

1. Drink a glass of warm water and eat an apple before every meal
2. Take a teaspoon of sesame seeds and a teaspoon of olive oil after every meal
3. Take 1 clove of garlic daily (Not on an empty stomach)
4. Drink water during main meals (No drinks below room temperature)
5. Drink as much water as possible during the day – stop drinking water two hours before bedtime (sip some water if thirsty). When drinking a lot of water make sure to also use salt to keep nutrients and minerals in your body
6. Use onions in your socks, ears and nose. They clean/purify the blood, help get rid of toxins and kill bacteria and germs and therefor help improve any kind of medical condition. Absorbed through the skin, onions act like an internal shampoo. You can also blend onions and add them to a foot- or hand bath or a full bath, this helps expel toxins and

waste from your body and all its systems and organs, cleansing your body down to cellular level.

7. Practice the new way of breathing and you will eventually do it as normal. Breathe through your nose slowly and make the breath as long as you can. Breathe out through your nose a little faster to expel the carbon dioxide.

8. Do not eat any meat from the pig. Pigs have no sweating mechanisms; hence all toxins are contained in the meat; this increases when the meat is heated.

THINGS TO AVOID

1. All pig/pork products, i.e. bacon, ham, pork, sausages, rashers, etc.
2. Smoking
3. Alcohol
4. Hot spicy foods
5. Oily greasy foods
6. Sweet/salty foods
7. Do not eat if you are not hungry
8. Do not eat for at least four hours before bedtime
9. Avoid too much RED meat and dairy products

RECIPES

NATURAL ANTIBIOTIC

(1) ½ an orange peel,

(2) ½ an apple;

(3) teaspoon of honey;

(4) 1 teaspoon of olive oil;

(5) 2-3 cloves of garlic;

(6) A pinch of black pepper;

(7) Drop of lemon juice;

(8) Drop of vinegar

Blend all the ingredients together.

You may have to add hot water to help make it into a thick liquid, which can be used as a drink or a spread. It can also be used as a salad dressing or a sauce over fish, chicken or meat. Take the Natural Antibiotic daily but especially in the winter months

CLEANSING DRINK

Fill a mug with boiling water and add …

(1) ½ teaspoon of salt

(2) A pinch of black pepper;

(3) A pinch of curry powder

(4) A Pinch of paprika powder

(5) A Pinch of turmeric

(6) A few drops of lemon juice

(7) A few drops of vinegar

(8) A few drops of olive oil

(9) The tip of a teaspoon of honey

Stir well and Enjoy.

Testimonials

East West Clinic Waterford City is a very popular place for health and spiritual wellbeing. Dheai explains how the structure of the body can be healed through acupuncture and to improve one's general health. He covers everything from the tips of your toes to the hair on your head. His book covers all aspects of health, it is an ideal guide for anyone wishing to improve their health and wellbeing, for a healthy life. Having met Dheai many years ago, I was overwhelmed by his knowledge and his awareness of the human body. I started using his philosophy in my own practice. Having gone to many of his lectures it is always an insight into reality.

John McGrath FHP DIP SAC MPS PRACT
Foot Health Clinic

It is with great pleasure that I congratulate Dheai on the publication of his first book. From his busy practices in Waterford and Templemore, Dheai treats each client from an Emotional, Physical, Structural and Functional aspect. Personally, I have greatly benefited from attending the East West Clinic, I believe early detection and intervention by Dheai has helped to save my health. I have also attended many of Dheai's lectures and workshops, and I have found them to be very informative, offering attendees a wonderful opportunity to gain a deeper understanding of the theory behind Dheai's therapy.

Eileen Kennedy. M.I.A.C.P.

Dheai Ilsaaid, a General Oriental Practitioner based in Waterford city Ireland, is the author of this book about Oriental Medicine. I have seen his interaction first hand over the last ten years with clients who benefit from an alternative approach to diagnosis and management than is provided by conventional Western medicine. He combines firstly an eagle eyed, carefully honed skill of clinic observation with a caring integrated approach to management which includes acupuncture, mobilisation, massage, mindfulness practices and exercise programmes delivered with a marvellous enthusiasm for, and appreciation of, the oriental perspective on the mind body spirit integration which he conveys to his clients. For many with musculoskeletal non-inflammatory conditions, his approach is exactly what they seek in a non-pharmaceutical based integrated option. Clearly this can be combined with the Western approach. His treatments are successful in alleviating pain and dysfunction in many. His enthusiasm for his subject, delivered with confidence and competence, allows the Eastern tradition of seven thousand years of observation and intervention be combined with a Western appreciation of our traditions and management options with significant benefit for the client accruing. Dheai has an excellent knowledge of anatomy, physiology and Eastern philosophy. This book gives knowledge of Yin and Yang and Qi and seeks to put them into a Western perspective. It is particularly strong in explaining how emotions play such a major part in our lives and health. His book gives an insight as to how the body manifests the trials and tribulations of the mind, how the Oriental practitioner diagnoses problems of his clients and how re-examination can confirm that his interventions suggested have been a success. I am happy to encourage people to get an insight into how East can synergise with West for the client's benefit.

Dr Darragh Foley-Nolan MD, Consultant Rheumatologist and Physician

DHEAI ILSAAID

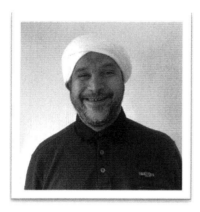

Dheai Ilsaaid opened his first practice in Ireland in 2004, catering only for football players. In 2005 Dheai opened the first East-West Clinic in Waterford City to the public, the second followed in 2011 in Templemore.

When Dheai isn't shouting at people to *"Mind The Step"*, he runs weekly Medical Yoga classes, gives regular Workshops and Seminars on Oriental Medicine and Eastern Philosophy and with the little free time he has left, he coaches the local football team.

MIND THE STEP